CHRIS SHELTON'S
EASY GUIDE TO
EMOTIONAL
WELL-BEING
WITH QIGONG

CHRIS SHELTON'S EASY GUIDE TO EMOTIONAL WELL-BEING WITH QIGONG

THIRD EDITION

CHRIS SHELTON

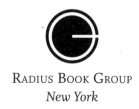

RADIUS BOOK GROUP
New York

Radius Book Group
A division of Diversion Publishing Corp.
www.radiusbookgroup.com

Radius Book Group and colophon are registered
trademarks of Diversion Publishing Corp.

For more information, email info@radiusbookgroup.com

Although the author and publisher have made every effort to ensure that the
information in this book was correct at press time, the author and publisher
do not assume and hereby disclaim any liability to any party for any loss,
damage, or disruption caused by errors or omissions, whether such errors
or omissions result from negligence, accident, or any other cause.

Neither the author nor the publisher assumes any responsibility or liability,
whatsoever, on behalf of the consumer or reader of this material. Any
perceived slight of any individual or organization is purely unintentional.

The resources in this book are provided for informational purposes only
and should not be used to replace the specialized training and professional
judgment of a health care or mental health care professional.

Neither the author nor the publisher can be held responsible for the use of the
information provided within this book. Please always consult a trained professional
before making any decision regarding treatment of yourself or others.

First Radius Book Group Edition: January 2025
Second Edition: July 2017
First Edition: September 2013
Paperback ISBN: 9781635768831
E-book ISBN: 9781635768855

Book design by Scribe Inc.
Cover design by Jen Huppert
Illustrations: Chris Shelton
Model: Shelby Bearschild & Nare Israelyan
Line and Copy Editor: Nichole Gates
Photographers: George Clark & Chris Schmauch
Book cover design: Joshua Orenstein & Chris Shelton
Graphic designer: Joshua Orenstein
Headshot: Greg Zabilski
Project Manager: Parisa Shelton

For more information, email news@sheltonqigong.com

Printed in the United States of America
3 5 7 9 10 8 6 4

■ ■ ■

EXTRA RESOURCES

To give you the best experience with this book, my team and I have created an online resource that includes my Five Element Questionnaire, as well as detailed descriptions of the different personality types.

You'll find a copy of these and the rest of your resources by scanning the QR code below or by visiting this website:

www.qigongforemotionalwellbeing.com

■ ■ ■

DEDICATION

When I wrote the first edition of this book in 2013, its primary purpose was to introduce people to the healing practices of Qigong and to give them tools to enhance their overall state of well-being. I explained how negative emotions affect different organs and manifest as inflammation and disease, and how these simple, time-tested practices can help one remove stagnant or stuck emotions and improve their quality of life. Since 2013, my team has been awarded government contracts to assist county employees by providing mental health resources and tools for overcoming stress. I've since had the honor of being a keynote speaker on the role negative emotions play in the formation of disease. In addition, I began to regularly communicate with trauma nurses and doctors, county supervisors, the Sheriff's Department, and social services. In 2015, thanks to Maria Shriver, I performed Qigong at the Special Olympics World Games. After that, the Special Olympics initiated a program called Healthy Athletes Strong Minds, where Parisa and I became clinical directors for Northern California and Nevada. In this program, we teach Qigong practices to the athletes, coaches, and their families to effectively deal with the stress of competition and, more importantly, to respond appropriately to bullying and conflict.

Throughout the years, I've witnessed the many ways emotional trauma shows up in the body and the lack of resources available to those struggling with mental health conditions. Mental and emotional disorders not only affect the person living with them but also have a ripple effect on friends and family who support or care for them. This ripple effect significantly impacts those left behind when an individual goes so far as to take their own life as a result of mental and emotional pain and suffering.

This hits particularly close to home, because on Thanksgiving morning, 2022, my best friend took his own life. Most who knew of this were under the impression that it was a sudden and random event. However, having been so close to him, he previously confided in me that the pharmaceuticals he had been prescribed a year-and-a-half prior were causing him to feel seriously depressed and have suicidal thoughts. He came to see me at the clinic and began following the advice I recommended, which largely involved incorporating Qigong practices into his daily life. He achieved a healthy and balanced state of mind for quite a while. Then, at one point, something shifted and he lost this momentum, choosing instead to return to old habits and prescription drugs that came with serious and dangerous side effects before, ultimately, ending his life.

This book is dedicated to those who struggle with mental illness and to others who have lost loved ones as a result of mental health issues. My hope is that the practices in this book will liberate you from mental anguish and suffering, allowing you to live the life God has designed for you so you may reach your fullest potential.

This book is also dedicated to my beautiful wife Parisa, who makes my world turn; to Mary Theresa, who went through the second edition with extra attention to detail; to Nichole Gates, who meticulously edited my second book, *Chris Shelton's Easy Guide to Fix Neck and Back Pain*, and now the third edition of this book; to the countless friends and family who support my mission of bringing Qigong to the world; and to my loyal students, who make the Work worthwhile. Thank you.

∎ ∎ ∎
CONTENTS

■ ■ ■

FOREWORD

Greetings!

I have been in the holistic health field for over 30 years. I am a gastronaut of sorts—an explorer of numerous pure diets and healing systems: vegetarianism, raw foods, superfood and superherb diets, ketogenic, intermittent and long fasting, wild foods, Native American herbalism, Amazonian shamanism, Ayurvedic medicine, Chinese medicine, and all kinds of mixtures thereof.

Through my exploration of diets, healing systems, and healthy lifestyles, I basically became an Indiana Jones type of character, writing books and traveling the world in search of exotic superfoods, healing systems, and herbal medicines. Over the years, I have been blessed with the tremendous honor of touching the lives of millions of people.

Two of my favorite people I met along my journey have been Chris and Parisa Shelton. They are like family to me and great teachers to me as well. I feel a special privilege in introducing you to this book: the third edition of *Chris Shelton's Easy Guide to Emotional Well-Being With Qigong.*

My first encounter with Chris Shelton's work was through a mutual friend, Eric the Trainer, Hollywood Physique Expert. Learning how Chris utilized ancient information for healing today really resonated with me. His approach is designed for everyday people. When I discovered his vast knowledge of health and healing, and the beautiful way he shared that knowledge, I knew the two of us would be lifelong friends.

Chris is dedicated to enhancing your quality of life. He is a people person. His work and this book are precious gems that I feel fortunate to have discovered, and I know you will feel the same—the information in these pages comes as a gift from a power greater than ourselves.

This book is great for the new student and the advanced student alike—all levels welcome. I have been studying this material for 30 years, and I still found many new angles and ideas in these pages, as well as many things I love to study and review again and again. Constant review of the fundamentals found in this book will assist both your healing journey and/or your work in the healing field.

In this book, you will find gentle and time-tested tools to activate ancient practices that reverse the aging process, slow down disease, and elevate mood along with emotions. By uncovering your Five Elements archetype and understanding your constitution, you will embark on a transformational journey toward improved mental clarity and emotional well-being.

What I love about this book is that it is accessible to all levels. Personally, I always had trouble learning the meridian system of Chinese medicine because the drawings and images were tough for me to follow; however, this book makes it easy for me!

This book is immediately useful! A perfect reference manual and a constant reminder of the miracle of the human body. The easy-to-activate techniques shared in these pages are a testament to Chris Shelton's expertise and dedication to empowering individuals to live healthier, more fulfilling lives.

The text is filled with gems of time-tested methods, honed over centuries, offering immediate relief and paving the way for long-term healing. You can find your way out of pain and despair and reach towards the heavens in harmony and inspiration.

May this information be a beacon of health, vitality, and transformation on your path to emotional well-being.

You can heal yourself. You can help others to heal themselves. And this wonderful book is a necessary instructional guide to make the magic happen faster! I was always taught: "When all else fails, read the instructions!" So here they are . . .

Have the best day ever!

David 'Avocado' Wolfe
Author, Nutritionist, Organic Farmer, Adventurer, World Traveler

■ ■ ■

INTRODUCTION

This book describes the theories and practices of specific exercises focused on balancing your body's energy. Although they originated in ancient China, these exercises are meant to benefit all people. The system as a whole is known as "Qigong." "Qi" refers to the life force energy that emanates within all things, material and non-material, and "gong" means work, or skill. Practicing the meditations and exercises described in this book will certainly give your Qi a boost, and you will finish feeling revitalized and refreshed, rather than worked-out and exhausted. Each day of practice will bring greater and greater benefits, gradually refining your health and vitality—your fundamental nature—as one would refine ore into gold.

This book began as a collection of handouts for a course I teach. I have included both those handouts and the text of accompanying lectures. Thus, it can serve either as a complete self-study guide for anyone who would like to explore the effects of this ancient and extraordinary system, or as a reference for those who have taken my course. No special equipment is required. The meditations and exercises are simple; you need only patience and perseverance to succeed.

The first section of the book (chapters 1–12) focuses on Classical Chinese medicine (CCM) principles of how the body functions and related practices. In Chinese medicine, we see the body as an intricate network of energy pathways. Each pathway is associated with particular functions and organs that can be influenced by distinct movements, sounds, and even thoughts. By practicing the meditations and exercises described in this book, you will learn to stimulate and harmonize the vital energy flow within your body. Examples of how these exercises have helped me, my family, and my clients are also included in the text.

The second section of the book (chapters 13–30) includes the Five Elements healing sounds and deeper cleansing exercises for strengthening your body and promoting emotional well-being. The following section (chapters 31–38) focuses on Five Elements principles as they apply to individuals. The Five Elements are expressed in a person's appearance and behavior. They can be used to diagnose disease as well as to enhance life. Emotions are a key component of overall health. This is why addressing emotional issues is absolutely critical in all that I teach and in my healing practice. The tools I have personally found useful in restoring emotional balance are also included in the text.

The final section (chapters 39–41) brings it all together. The Qigong practices, Yin and Yang Typology Questionnaire, application of Five Elements principles, and emotional work comprise an effective, comprehensive means of understanding your fundamental nature and refining your Qi, thereby allowing you to realize your full potential as a human being.

Personal History

My path to Qigong began at age 19 after two heart attacks from drug use and a near-paralyzing back injury from a bad kick in Tae Kwon Do. It is no exaggeration when I say Qigong saved my life.

I was a rebellious and arrogant teenager with an explosive temper. My friends were doing drugs, so I thought, "Hey, why not me too?" I felt invincible—that is, until I ended up in the emergency room from a drug overdose. Finally, it became clear that continuing on my present course would put me either in prison or the grave. I decided that taking up Tae Kwon Do was my ticket to a new life. I trained hard, enjoying the vigorous workouts and the challenge of going up against an opponent until one night, while training for a tournament, I was accidentally kicked in the back. The blow left me almost paralyzed.

For the first time in my life, I experienced helplessness. I couldn't wipe myself in the bathroom or put on my shoes and socks. From an X-ray of my back, a chiropractor confirmed what the western doctors had told me: if I wasn't careful, the injury could paralyze me from the waist down. She referred me to a massage therapist who was also a martial artist. While he worked on me, he taught me about Qi. As a 21-year-old boy, I was convinced that this "Qi" was some kind of hocus-pocus. My Tae Kwon Do instructors had talked about "Ki," but only in terms of the sound you make at the moment you throw a punch or kick. What my future teacher was describing seemed entirely different. He told me that, yes, Qi could be used for martial arts, but it also could be used to heal the body.

Intrigued, impressed by his sincerity, and feeling better, I started taking Qigong classes. At that time, because of my years of drug use, I had kidney and liver problems, sinusitis, and digestive problems. The digestive problems were so severe that within an hour of eating, I was nauseated. I survived on a variety of antacids and antibiotics. So, I started practicing Qigong. I was doing the guided meditations and gentle movement practices regularly, but without real dedication. I was really just "going through the motions," as they say. Even so, after some time—perhaps six months or a year—I realized that my health ailments had gone away. I was breathing easily and could eat without feeling sick to my stomach! Similarly, two women in my Qigong class, one with arthritis and the other with asthma, reported that their conditions had almost completely resolved by the end of that same year.

As my internal organs recovered, so did my back. Western doctors went from telling me I would never walk again to saying I would be able to walk but could never train again. They then said I would be able to train, but could never fight again. Proving them wrong, I continued to compete in Kung Fu and kickboxing tournaments until the age of 40.

What Is Qi?

Even after recovering and experiencing the power of these deceptively simple exercises, I still did not fully understand what Qi was or how this miracle had occurred. All I knew was there was something to it. Somehow, it worked. Now, after more than 20 years of practicing and working with Qi, I have more of an appreciation of what it is and can offer the following description.

According to Chinese medicine, Qi is the energy that creates, infuses, and sustains the universe and, thus, life. It is said to be present in inanimate objects, like rocks, as well as living things, like plants and animals, and the subtle states of immaterial things, like air, light, sound, and thought. There are many different forms of Qi.

When Qi is strong and coherent, life flourishes. Conversely, if Qi becomes stagnant, deficient, or scattered, this opens the door to disease and, ultimately, death. Qigong is a means of working with, cultivating, and developing your personal Qi. In other words, it is a method for maintaining your vital life force. It is not based on belief; you do not have to believe in it for it to work. The concept of Qi is at the heart of Classical Chinese Medicine (CCM), and Qigong-type exercises are as old as the medicine itself. The fact that this medicine has been around for more than 5,000 years is, in itself, evidence that it works. History has shown that anything fake or false inevitably reveals its flaws over time and is discarded. (I would like to add that, to do Qigong, you do not have to wear fancy silk pajamas or a cloak.)

Curative Qigong® is a program I created based on the Five Elements, Qigong, Tong-style Acupuncture, and Classical Chinese Medicine. It is an integrated approach to healthcare that works with the environment, emotions, and physical body to understand pathology and how this affects the proper functioning of the organs and organism as a whole, eventually showing up as disease. The course combines sensitivity training and listening techniques of Qigong with palpation and tonification or dredging of acupoints, channels, collateral channels, and organ systems to bring about homeostasis and reverse the process of chronic pain and disease.

How does Qigong work? Qi flows in specific pathways within the body called meridians. Each meridian is associated with a particular organ, for the most part corresponding to the anatomical organs according to western medicine.

Meridians can be compared to rivers and the internal organs to lakes that are supplied and drained by these rivers. Thus, just as in nature, when there is not enough water flowing in a river, the lake it feeds will eventually dry out, adversely affecting the surrounding environment and all related ecosystems. Conversely, when too much water flows, the lake will overflow its boundaries. Using this metaphor, we can see that the purpose of Qigong is to balance and harmonize the rivers and lakes of the body, so they may function at their peak capacity.

Beauty Beyond the Physical

According to Chinese medicine, the two leading causes of disease are negative emotions and diet. Diet and emotions influence the body differently, but ultimately interact. Diet supplies the physical substance from which the body continually recreates itself. Emotions, too, are a kind of diet, because they determine the quality of the subtle energies of the body which control organ function. Based on observations made by ancient Chinese doctors over centuries, we know that the internal organs each store different negative emotions, and when these emotions are held or expressed inappropriately, the proper functioning of related organs becomes disrupted, sometimes causing fatal health problems. Each organ system stores different kinds of energy and is damaged by excesses or deficiencies of these particular energies. In Curative Qigong®, we understand that these internal organs are interrelated, such that a dysfunction of one can eventually lead to dysfunction in another. Thus, in clinical practice, a Curative Qigong® practitioner can work backward from the disease that is manifesting to the emotional toxins present in order to find the true root of a condition.

Another aspect of emotional health is one's attitude toward aging and beauty. So often nowadays, we see people focused on their external beauty, having surgery or liposuction and using techniques like Botox. Curative Qigong® in general and Qigong in particular address this issue from two standpoints. First, it tackles the inherent attitude. Why is a person so concerned about their appearance? Is there fear or hatred within? Exploring these questions can be very important. When your organs are in harmony, you will feel so good—enjoying your life, family, and work—that you will not have time for such negative thoughts. Second, it asks you to reassess what beauty means, in a deeper sense. When your organs, including your skin, are functioning properly, not storing negative emotions or toxic digestive waste, you will radiate health—and beauty—at any age.

Simple Practices, Profound Results

To our western minds, it seems incredible that these simple movements and meditations can have such profound effects. No surgery? Supplements? Drugs? But it's true. You can experience this yourself. Indeed, one of the values of Qigong is that you will gradually become your own doctor. Doing these practices will put you in touch with your body in subtle ways. You will develop a sensitivity to both the emotional and physical conditions present in your body. Eventually, you will be able to detect disease before it sets in. You will recognize the first signs of imbalance, and with the meditations and exercises described in this book, you will have the tools to correct them.

If you have a hard time accepting the concept of Qi or theories about how it works, then—as I did in the beginning—ignore it all! Just do the exercises. Based on the successful experiences of countless generations of people who have used these exercises and passed them down to us, give them a try. Observe carefully; the body has its own wisdom as to how and when it heals. You may be surprised by what changes, and it may not happen as you expect. Simply, practice consistently. Over time, you will experience greater vitality, health, and mental well-being.

The journey of a thousand miles begins with a single step. Take that step and enjoy the journey!

Chris Shelton
January 2025
Burbank, CA

■ ■ ■

HOW TO USE THIS BOOK

If you are new to Chinese medical theories, I recommend you start at the beginning and work through each chapter, just as though you were taking my course. The information in each chapter corresponds to a lesson of my course, each building on the previous one. There are many terms and concepts that are specific to Chinese; I have tried to explain each new one when I use it. While you may have a particular health concern that you want to address—arthritis, high blood pressure, depression, or anxiety, for example—the body is still a coherent and complete system. What affects one part will affect the body as a whole. As you work through the book, you will become acquainted with how the Chinese conceive of these body parts working in unison and, consequently, how affecting one will impact another. Thus, when you address your issue (or those of your clients if you are a practitioner), you will also be aware of changes elsewhere in the body, so you can maintain good overall health.

    If you are familiar with Chinese medical theories and perhaps other forms of Qigong, you may be able to go directly to the sections that interest you. Nevertheless, I do recommend you at least skim through the other sections, if only for review. Hopefully, you will find some new kernel of knowledge that will increase and deepen your understanding. In any case, remember that the body is a coherent whole, and we must keep the big picture in mind as we work on one aspect of it.

    For everyone, chapter 30 provides suggestions for establishing a regular practice. Regularity is important; the body has rhythms just as the cosmos do. Patience and persistence are important, because results may come slowly, especially at first. The more you practice, the more quickly you will experience results; however, even more important than the amount of time you spend is the quality of that time. Your undistracted attention is absolutely critical. In the beginning, you may simply be learning to stay focused; that is good. As in any mindfulness training, keep trying (without disappointment or frustration), and your body will respond; your Qi will flourish.

A note about capitalization: if the text refers to the actual physical organ, the word will be lowercase. If it refers to the energetic qualities of the organ system, the word will be capitalized.

· CHAPTER 1 ·

FOUNDATIONS

People know when they are sick; they also know how they feel when they are well. This is a matter of awareness of what the Chinese call "Qi." The practice of Qigong (pronounced chee-gong) focuses on refining this awareness. Which part of the body is sick? What is wrong with the Qi? Is it stuck? Is there too much or too little? Through the meditations and exercises of Qigong, we can answer these questions and learn how to remedy problems. By practicing them, we can experience and create vibrant health.

Just as we know in our bodies when something is not quite right, we can also feel differences in the weather as well as in people, even before they speak. All of this awareness involves energy. The ancient Chinese devised a universal system to describe the various forms of energy, not only in the human body and in the weather, but also in space (in landscape and geography), and over time (in history and astrology). By understanding that everything in the cosmos is an expression of Qi, from the material to the insubstantial, one can glimpse the ultimate truth of the universe and come to a deep understanding and appreciation of the natural world, including one's own true nature.

The core text of Chinese philosophy is the I Ching, or Book of Changes. Its basic premise is that energy evolves from the unmanifest to the manifest realm. These manifestations may be broadly described as Yin and Yang. Beyond Yin and Yang, all manifestations may be more precisely (but still generally) described in terms of the Five Elements. And beyond those, there are the "ten thousand things," all of which are permutations of these broader concepts.

Health is an expression of the smooth flow of life-giving Qi in the body. Disease manifests when the flow of Qi is blocked or stagnant, or when there is too much or too little. Physical and mental exercises can clear blockage, dissolve stagnation, reduce excess, and supplement deficiency. I will use the terms "excess" and "deficiency" throughout this text as they are used in CCM and Curative Qigong®. They describe conditions in which there is too much of something, i.e., when an organ is hyperactive, or when there is too little, i.e., the organ is weak or hypoactive.

In these chapters, you will learn how to interpret the signs and signals of the body in terms of these patterns as well as how to correct and improve the flow of Qi. That is the practice and purpose of Qigong. It can benefit you as well as your clients, if you are a practitioner.

Centers of Energy: The Tan Tiens

Three is a number often used to describe or simplify the complexity of our human experience. In Christianity, the aspects of God are described as Father, Son, and Holy Ghost. In Chinese metaphysics, the components of the universe are described as Heaven, Earth, and Man. In the human body, CCM and Curative Qigong® sees three "Tan Tiens" (pronounced dahn tee-ENS), or energy centers, that correspond to the physical, emotional/mental, and spiritual aspects of a person's being. These vital energy centers are located along the midline of the body and store energy much in the way batteries do.

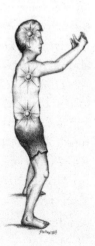

UPPER

The upper Tan Tien relates to our spiritual being. It roughly comprises the upper, anterior portion of the skull, and is found in the region of what is commonly referred to as the third eye. In western medicine, the upper Tan Tien corresponds to the Central Nervous System (CNS) which, through nerve impulses, controls the functions of all organs.

MIDDLE

The middle Tan Tien relates to our mental/emotional state and is associated with the Heart center in the middle of the chest.

LOWER

The lower Tan Tien relates to the physical aspect of our being and is located about an inch below the navel, in the center of the body. This is the area most people refer to when they speak of the Tan Tien. As all physical energy is stored and used from this region, we will refer to it often in our Qigong practices.

Basic Guidelines for Practicing Qigong

PRACTICAL ASPECTS

The goal of Qigong is to harmonize and develop your energy. If you do what you can to harmonize the physical aspects of the practice—your body and the environment—you will achieve your goal more quickly and to a much greater extent. When your body and mind are nourished, rested, calm, and relaxed, you will be in a natural state of equilibrium. A smooth flow of vigorous Qi will be expressed through your health and vitality.

TIME AND PLACE

1. Practice in a clean, well-ventilated place.

2. Choose a time and place where you will not be disturbed.

3. Practice regularly—ideally in the same place and time.

4. Avoid eating meals 30 to 60 minutes before practice. Yet, do not practice when hungry. Your body should feel comfortable and relaxed.

5. If you do heavy anaerobic exercise, like weightlifting, on a day you practice Qigong, be sure to stretch before and after to keep the meridians open.

LIFESTYLE

- ☯ Get proper rest and sleep.

- ☯ Avoid drinks that are ice cold.

- ☯ Avoid drugs and alcohol.

- ☯ Avoid fatty, greasy, sugary, and processed foods.

- ☯ Moderate your sexual activity.

- ☯ For women: Stop practice during your monthly period, or, if you do practice, shift your focus to the middle Tan Tien.

The Three Regulations

BREATH

Breathing should be natural, slow, smooth, even, and deep. Allow the abdomen to relax so that it rises with each inhalation and falls with each exhalation. Do not use force. At the end of each exhalation, the body will naturally initiate inhalation. Always breathe through your nose to better regulate the flow of Qi.

MIND

Like the breath, the mind should be relaxed. At the same time, it needs to be focused, because visualization is used in most of the meditations, and the mind will be used to guide Qi. Balance relaxation with alert curiosity as it relates to what is happening in your body. With firm but gentle determination, maintain your attention and intention.

WUJI POSTURE

Proper body alignment provides the ways and means for smooth energetic flow. In Tai Ji and Qigong, this proper body alignment is called Wuji Posture, where "wu" means "none," and "ji" (the same *ji* of Tai Ji, or Tai Chi) means "extreme." Hence, this is the way of standing that has no extremes. It is sometimes called the "emptiness" posture. It is commonly used for beginning and ending movements and can also be used alone as a standing meditation. Here are steps to achieving the correct Wuji Posture:

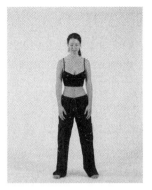
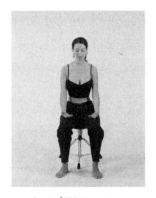

Standing Wuji posture   *Seated Wuji posture*

Wuji Posture

1. Stand with your feet approximately shoulder-width apart, toes pointing straight ahead.

2. Allow your knees to relax; do not lock them.

3. Tuck the tip of the sacrum under, as if sitting down. This subtle movement lengthens the spine and opens the Gate of Life point, or Ming Men, located on the spine opposite the navel.

4. Drop the shoulders and allow them to spread like wings, widening the back.

5. Tuck the chin and imagine the top of your head (the Crown Point) being pulled upward.

6. Feel your weight pressing down through the balls of the feet to stimulate the Kidney meridian.

7. Breathe slowly, smoothly, evenly, and deeply, inhaling and exhaling like a balloon through your lower abdominal region.

8. Empty your mind.

9. Place the tip of the tongue on the roof of the mouth behind the teeth, as if saying "nnnn."

As mind, breath, and body become calm and centered through these three regulations, notice yourself becoming more alert. This is the flow of Qi.

Pulling Down the Heavens

The practice of Pulling Down the Heavens is a staple of Qigong. I recommend doing it before and after every exercise. It is a simple, sweeping movement.

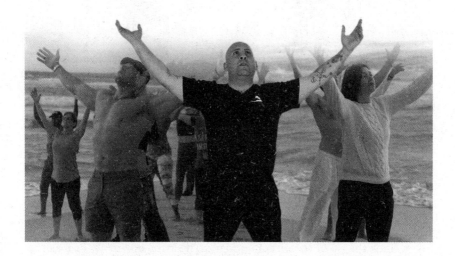

1. Begin in Wuji posture. As you inhale, raise, or float, your arms wide to the side, palms up and gently curved.

2. At the top of your reach, as you begin to exhale, turn your palms over and bring the arms down, with elbows bent and palms parallel facing you, passing in front of your face, then your abdomen.

3. Do this three times in a continuous sweeping motion. On the first sweep, you might picture pure white light flowing down the outside of your body. On the second, imagine pure white light flowing through the inside of your body, and on the third, imagine this white light flowing both within and all around you—suffusing your entire body.

4. End the sequence by returning to Wuji posture.

White Pearl Meditation

This meditation will help ground your energy as well as restore your vitality; it specifically enhances Kidney Essence, which will be discussed in chapter 10. It is helpful anytime you feel depleted and is also good as a basic daily practice. The White Pearl Meditation is available on music streaming platforms.

1. Assume Wuji posture; remember the Three Regulations of mind, breath, and posture. Check your alignment from head to toe and look for any tension. Relax down the body—front, back, and center.

2. Pull Down the Heavens three times.

3. Place your hands on the lower Tan Tien, just below the navel on the abdomen.

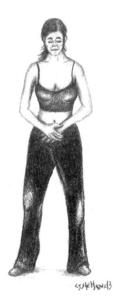

4. With eyes closed, breathe through the nose and into the lower Tan Tien. Keep your breath long, smooth, even, and deep. Allow and feel the breath expanding the abdomen to the front, back, left, and right simultaneously. This expansion and contraction will fill the lower Tan Tien with breath and Qi.

5. Imagine your lower Tan Tien as a white luminescent pearl of incredible beauty. As you breathe, the energy from the heavens and your tissues fills the lower Tan Tien. See and feel this

pearl becoming brighter and denser with each inhalation and exhalation.

6. Now use this energy to restore the "battery" of your own energy system, the Kidneys. As you inhale, see and feel the pearl expand with pure, luminous white light. As you exhale, see and feel the energy from the pearl fill and restore the left and right kidneys.

7. Continue this breathing pattern for 10 to 15 minutes.

8. Release the hands and open the eyes.

9. To finish, Pull Down the Heavens three more times.

NOTES

1. In step 5, you may place your hands on your abdomen. You might feel a warmth around your waist, as this corresponds to the Belt Vessel (an Extraordinary Meridian).

2. The most common error people make in doing this exercise is not pulling the breath down deeply enough. If you don't pull it down into the abdomen—that is, if you breathe only into the chest—you may experience gas and discomfort in your stomach.

3. In breathing, feel your lower abdomen (one inch below the navel, roughly corresponding to the lower Tan Tien) expand in all directions—front and back, side to side. This means it is totally relaxed. (Actually, it is good to breathe like this all day long.)

4. While best in the Wuji standing posture, the White Pearl Meditation can also be done sitting or lying down. If sitting, be sure to press the Crown Point of the head up. In both cases, remember to touch the tip of the tongue to the upper palate of your mouth, behind the teeth. If you are tired, it is better to sit and perform the meditation than to not do it at all.

5. This is a good general practice and is beneficial after any other daily routine or meditation.

General Comment

No matter how simple a practice may seem, it can have a profound effect. If you do not feel anything at first, do not worry that nothing is happening, especially in the early stages when you may not be very sensitive. Maintain your grounding, proper posture, sincere intention, and focused attention. With patience and perseverance, you will certainly make progress.

· CHAPTER 2 ·

THE NATURE OF QI

In Chinese metaphysics, Qi is the subtle energy that creates, sustains, activates, and animates the universe. As stated previously, it is said to be present in inanimate objects, like rocks, as well as in living things, like plants and animals, and in the subtle states of immaterial things, like air, light, sound, and thought. It is also said to have different qualities, or to be of different types; some of these are positive and nurturing for living beings, while others may be negative and destructive.

In our bodies, Qi can be subdivided in different ways. At conception, there are four influences present. One of which is Heavenly Qi, the basis of human consciousness, the natural vitality of the sperm and egg of the parents, and the energy of the time, place, and environment during conception. This is somewhat comparable to the western concept of genetics.

Prenatal Qi is the general name for the energy you were born with and is expressed in Kidney Qi. In other words, according to Chinese medicine, your constitution is expressed through the energy of your Kidneys, which we will discuss later. If your parents and ancestors were healthy, you are likely to be healthy as well.

After birth, you are nourished by what the Chinese call Postnatal Qi, which is derived from the Qi of the food you eat and the air you breathe. All of these energies are part of our overall Qi. The quality of each individual component contributes to the total state of your health. Essentially, when Qi is strong, flowing, and coherent, life will flourish.

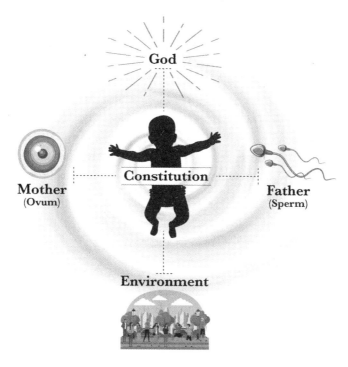

Mother (Ovum) · God · Constitution · Father (Sperm) · Environment

In summary, a person basically lives on two sources of energy: Prenatal Qi, the amount and quality of which was fixed at conception, and Postnatal Qi, which is somewhat under one's control. The more you conserve your Prenatal Qi, the longer you will live and the better the quality of your life will be. This means the stronger your Postnatal Qi, the less you will use up your supply of Prenatal Qi. In other words, if you eat well, breathe clean air, and live in a healthy environment, you will thrive on Postnatal Qi. But if you eat fast food, live erratically, or indulge in anger and anxiety, without sufficient Postnatal Qi, your body will use Prenatal Qi in its place, ultimately degrading and shortening your lifespan. Whenever your Qi becomes stagnant, deficient, or scattered, it opens the door to disease and, ultimately, death.

The purpose of regular Qigong practice is to harmonize and nurture your Qi. The first step is learning to feel Qi present within the body. We must become aware of what is happening in our bodies—especially in individual organ systems. This awareness does not come overnight; developing it is a lifelong practice. But even in the beginning, you should get a flash of it, a sense of the possibilities. Then, through meditations and exercises, with steady determination and regular practice, you can nurture that flash of light until it becomes a beacon. Once you are more aware, you can take the second step, which is to act appropriately. This course will give you exercises to develop your sensitivity to Qi and the methods you need to balance any disharmony that may arise.

Interestingly, as you become more aware of what is happening within your body, you will also become more sensitive to the Qi all around you, in the environment and in other beings—people, animals, and plants. As your sensitivity grows, your intuition and psychic ability will grow as well. You will then have the chance to improve your health on all levels. All Qi is connected.

Qi Clearing Exercises

The following three Body Awakening Exercises are another foundation of my Qigong practice. I recommend doing these before any Qigong session to bring your body and mind together in a centered state and to loosen the body, allowing for the free flow of Qi. It will make all of your subsequent practices more effective.

PRELIMINARY

1. Assume Wuji posture, remembering the Three Regulations.

2. Pull Down the Heavens three times.

TOSSING THE STONE

1. From Wuji posture, lift your arms out to the side until they are shoulder height, palms down (in a "T" position). Inhale.

2. As you exhale, turn your upper torso to one side and swing the opposite arm, palm up (as though tossing a stone) while the other arm swings behind you.

3. Inhale as you return to the "T" position.

4. As you exhale, repeat on the other side. In other words, if you turn to the right, your left arm will swing in front and to the right as though tossing a stone, while your right arm will swing behind you.

5. Repeat in a continuous rhythm, synchronized with your breathing, first one side then the other. Do this 3 to 9 times on each side.

6. End by Pulling Down the Heavens three times.

THE HEEL DROP

1. From Wuji posture, begin lightly bouncing on the balls of your feet.

2. As you bounce, mentally visit each major joint of your body and release any tension there. Picture the tension descending down and out of the body. Start with your ankles and move up to the knees, then the hips, ending at the Heart center. Next, move to the fingers and travel up the arms, through the wrists, elbows, and shoulders, ending at the neck.

3. Stop bouncing. Imagine gold light rising through your body.

4. Rise up on the balls of your feet and inhale, pulling the light up to and beyond the top of your head. Then quickly and sharply drop to your heels, releasing all tension into the earth.

5. Repeat the sequence 3 to 9 times.

6. End by Pulling Down the Heavens three times.

SHAKING THE TREE VERSION 1

1. From Wuji posture, raise your arms out in front of you, parallel, about shoulder height.

2. Inhale while making loose fists, as though hauling something at the end of a rope.

3. Exhale as you pull your hands alternately to your chest in a flowing motion, shaking your arms and upper torso, down through the body.

4. Repeat continuously, starting with slow, large movements, each successive one faster and smaller as your hands reach your chest.

5. Immediately shake your entire body from head to toe. The more relaxed you are, the more you will feel the vibration throughout your whole body, including within your internal organs.

6. Repeat the exercise 3 to 9 times.

7. End by Pulling Down the Heavens three times.

SHAKING THE TREE VERSION 2

1. From Wuji posture, start with your hands at your sides.

2. Inhale. While relaxing the hands, prepare to shake from head to toe.

3. Exhale as you vigorously begin to shake from the fingers, up the hands, and into the arms in rapid waves. Let the shake ripple all the way up to the top of the head, then down to the bottoms of the feet.

4. Repeat continuously, starting at the fingertips with small shaking movements that grow into larger, more rapid ones as the movement travels up the arms to the top of the head then down to the feet, with arms and hands remaining at your sides.

5. The more relaxed you are, the more you will feel the vibration throughout your whole body, including within your internal organs.

6. Repeat the exercise 3 to 9 times.

7. End by Pulling Down the Heavens three times.

Center and Balance Meditation

The Center and Balance Meditation is the basic exercise for developing a relationship with your own body as well as with the cosmic energies of Heaven and Earth. It asks you to be present in the now, in your body and not in your head. The meditation is also available on music streaming platforms.

1. Start with the Three Regulations: steady breath, relaxed mind, Wuji posture (feet shoulder-width apart, shoulders relaxed, tailbone tucked, Crown Point rising).

2. Focus your attention on the front of your forehead in between the eyebrows. Imagine warm oil melting down the front of your body, covering everything in its path. Feel this oil absorbing impurities, leaving your cells clean and vibrant. Once the oil reaches your feet, feel it run off and down deep into the ground.

3. Now focus on the back of your head. Imagine smooth, warm oil flowing down the whole backside of your body. Feel it run down the back as you did the front. Visualize this warm oil covering and cleansing every cell and tissue of your body, again flowing off your feet, deep into the earth.

4. Next, focus your attention on the top of the head at what is called the Crown Point (GV 20) in Chinese medicine. Take a moment to connect with your higher power. Imagine a white light from Heaven entering the Crown Point and flowing down through the body, cleansing the internal organs. Imagine this white light permeating down to the cellular level. Visualize it going through the head, down your spine, abdomen, and legs, out of the feet, and deep into the ground.

5. Imagine that your feet are melting into the earth, leaving you standing in a sea of liquid energy about the height of your ankles.

6. Visualize roots growing down from the centers of your feet, the Bubbling Well (KI 1) point in Chinese medicine. These roots connect deep into the earth, twice the height of the body. This will give you a strong connection with both Heaven and Earth.

7. Inhale, imagining energy from the Earth going up the roots and through your legs, expanding into your lower Tan Tien. Exhale as you imagine the energy going back down into the ground. Repeat this over and over, filling up the entire lower abdomen then releasing the energy down into the earth.

8. End by spreading both arms out to the sides, raising them up over your head, and bringing them down in front, finally resting your palms on top of one another over your lower abdomen.

CHAPTER 3

THE MERIDIAN SYSTEM

The word meridian, as used in Chinese medicine, entered the English language as a French translation of the Chinese medical term, Jing Luo. "Jing" means to go through or a thread in fabric, "luo" means something that connects or attaches, like a net.

Meridians are the channels, or pathways, that carry Qi throughout the body. They are different from physical blood vessels; instead, they are an invisible network of subtle energy pathways. In the meridian system, these channels represent a kind of informational network. Qi moves along them, connecting all of the organs as well as the interior and exterior of the body. The amount and quality of the flow of energy along these pathways determines the health of the body; deficiency, excess, stagnation, and blockage are the typical problems that may arise. The various therapies of Chinese medicine address these problems at specific points based on the details of the meridian system.

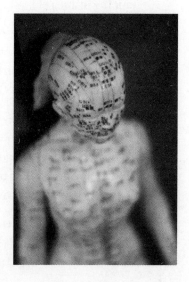

The meridian system of CCM and Curative Qigong® comprises twelve Regular Meridians and eight Extraordinary Meridians. The Extraordinary

Meridians, or Vessels, are actually part of the Regular Meridians and will be covered later.

The Regular Meridians are named according to the major organs of the body. Each meridian is a channel of energy associated with a particular organ; the energy runs between points where the flow can be influenced.

Regular Meridians function in Yin Yang pairs. The meaning of Yin and Yang will be explained in the next chapter. For now, simply think of Yin Yang components as being closely related, like masculine and feminine. Yin meridians are located on the inner aspects of the body; in them, Qi flows upward. Yang meridians are located on the outer aspects of the body where Qi flows downward. Each pair corresponds to one of the Five Elements, another set of concepts that will be explained later in chapter 6. The main point to understand for now is that Qi flows through the body in particular pathways called meridians. These meridians function in pairs, and each pair is associated with certain qualities and characteristics that are true both in the body and in nature.

The Twelve Meridians in Pairs According to the Five Elements

Element	FIRE	EARTH	METAL	WATER	WOOD	(Extra FIRE)
YIN	Heart	Spleen	Lungs	Kidney	Liver	Pericardium*
YANG	Small Intestine	Stomach	Large Intestine	Urinary Bladder	Gallbladder	Triple Burner*

The Pericardium is the tissue surrounding the heart, while the Triple Burner is a conceptual organ unique to the Chinese medical system. These will be described in a later chapter.

Brushing the Meridians

In this practice, we will use our hands to trace the meridians. This should harmonize and stimulate the flow of Qi. We will start by moving upward along the Yin meridians (inward sides of the body and limbs) as we inhale, and downward along the Yang meridians (outward sides of the body and limbs) as we exhale. Use a flat hand, palm facing the body. You may actually touch the body, or you may keep the hand just above the skin. The type of clothing you are wearing doesn't matter. Move at a speed consistent with your breath.

PRELIMINARY

1. Start with the Three Regulations: steady breath, relaxed mind, Wuji posture (feet shoulder-width apart, shoulders relaxed, tailbone tucked, Crown Point rising).

2. Pull Down the Heavens three times. You may lightly bounce to relax and loosen the body.

UPPER BODY

3. Begin with arms out to the side in a "T" position.

4. As you inhale, bring the hands together in front of the body, and draw each hand up the opposite arm. That is, the right hand moves up the outside of the left arm while the left hand moves up the outside of the right arm.

5. At the shoulder, continue moving the hands up the sides of the head (arms will be crossed).

6. As you reach the top of the head, allow the hands to uncross.

7. Exhale as you let the hands flow naturally down the sides of the body. Bending at the waist, continue to brush down the outside of the legs.

8. Roll up onto the balls of your feet as you flick your hands outward and say "SHUU" (shh-ooo), releasing your breath with a sharp exhalation while dropping your heels down. Imagine you are throwing any negative energy you have collected out of your hands and into the earth.

LOWER BODY

9. Next, lean over and put your hands on your ankles, left hand on left instep and right hand on right instep. As you inhale, move your hands up the inside of your legs toward the groin.

10. Cross your hands then move up along the abdomen and into the armpits.

11. Exhale. As you do, draw each hand down the opposite arm on the inside of the forearms until you pull your hands apart, palms facing each other.

12. Repeat from Step 1.

13. To end the practice, Pull Down the Heavens three times.

NOTES

1. Chinese texts recommend repeating this exercise 9 to 36 times (in multiples of 9, which is a harmonic number).

2. You can perform this practice using cupped hands to gently tap or pat along the meridian pathway rather than brushing. Remember to tap down the Yang meridians on the outer aspects of the body and up the Yin meridians along the inner aspects. Firmly pat with conviction to stimulate the flow of energy.

3. You can also do this exercise on other people using brushing or tapping. Either way, it should be an enjoyable and invigorating experience.

4. This is a good practice for anyone feeling physically "tight" or tense, because it stimulates the nerves and improves blood circulation.

5. This is also a good practice when you feel a cold or flu coming on, or when you sense any other imbalance in your energy. It should quickly restore inner harmony.

Feeling Bad Can Be Good

Do not expect to always feel good immediately after doing Qigong. By harmonizing energy flow, you are forcing issues to resolve themselves, and sometimes this can be uncomfortable. The practice is safe; continue, but perhaps more gently or slowly. Eventually, you should feel much better than before. You will not always know why—and knowing why doesn't really matter—but, in the long run, in my experience, you will definitely feel better.

· CHAPTER 4 ·

YIN AND YANG OF THE ORGANS

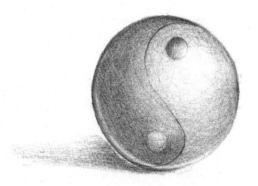

The philosophical concept of Yin and Yang is based on the understanding of relativity. Although fundamental to Chinese philosophy, the concept is foreign to western philosophical ideas. Historically, western philosophy has often employed absolutes in an attempt to determine what is true and not true. By contrast, Chinese philosophy is rooted in *relative* relationships, and these relationships are described using Yin and Yang. Just as something is big or small relative to what it is compared to; similarly, something is Yin or Yang relative to comparison with other things.

Heaven and Earth relate to Yang and Yin. Heaven embodies the active and dynamic characteristics of Yang while Earth's supportive foundation reflects Yin qualities. Together, they comprise the first division of Wuji, which refers to the divine realm out of which all things arise. Words cannot describe but only point to the magnitude, emptiness, and nothingness of the divine realm. This essence is what we attempt to achieve when standing in Wuji posture.

Yin and Yang have been at the forefront of Chinese philosophy for centuries. To understand Yin Yang principles, it is necessary to grasp the concept that everything is not what it seems. One must come to realize that every phenomenon in the multi-universe is an expression of Qi and is both itself and its contrary at the same time. The root of Yin is within Yang, and the root of Yang is within Yin.

Yin and Yang are, in essence, an expression of duality that we see, feel, and experience at all times. Together, they act as a language that describes the alternation and fluctuation of all things, at any moment in time. Every phenomenon in the multi-universe is an interchange of the cyclical movement of Yin and Yang. It is the underlying motivating force behind change, transformation, and restoration. Through studying this universal concept of balanced opposites, we realize that all things are always in a stage of flux and movement and that nothing exists in a static state of 50/50.

In ancient times, Yin and Yang were first described as two sides of a hill; one dark, the other light; one cool, the other hot. This accompanied the observation that every earthly phenomenon is constantly cycling between two opposing polarities; night becomes day, which again becomes night. Yet each end of the polarity is not in opposition to, but rather a part of, the whole to which its counterpart belongs.

Yin and Yang are, at the same time, both opposites and complements of one another. Qualities that are more active, bright, and expansive are relatively more Yang than those which are quiet, dark, or contracting, Yin traits. Furthermore, as part of an ongoing cyclical exchange between the two, Yin contains the root of Yang, and Yang the root of Yin. At its extreme, the one will even give rise to the other. For example, a period of intense, frantic activity (Yang) will often lead to a collapse of Yin, prompting the body to seek balance by shifting toward rest and recovery, Yin qualities. Yin and Yang are interdependent by definition and are constantly interchanging, one into the other. If you think about it, the body is a perfect reflection of the Tai Chi, or Yin Yang, symbol because the seed of Yin is present in Yang, and vice versa.

Here is a quick history of the discovery of these universal forces. The earliest origin of Yin and Yang is said to have come from ancient Chinese farmers who were seen as sages, wise individuals known for possessing deep wisdom and insight. Through their regular interaction with the environment, they observed the cyclical nature of seasonal changes, night and day, plant growth cycles, and weather patterns, all reflecting Yin Yang qualities. This led to the earliest observation that there are two opposed and balanced forces that correspond to every earthly phenomenon. This concept was then expanded to encompass the universal flow of these same energies.

The ancient sages conceived of Heaven (Yang) as a round vault and Earth (Yin) as flat. Therefore, Yang is represented by a circle, while a square is used to symbolize Yin. They concluded that Heavenly Yang contains the sun, moon, and stars (the basis for the Chinese lunar calendar) and relates to Earthly Yin which is responsible for time, earth, and space.

As the sun rises in the east and sets in the west, the direction of east is associated with Yang while west is considered Yin. In early Chinese cosmology, compass direction was oriented toward the south magnetic pole of the Earth, therefore making left (east) Yang, and right (west) Yin. There is some conflicting information pertaining to the right and left sides of the body and their association with Yin or Yang. From our studies, the left, Yang, side of the body and the right, Yin, side are based upon the natural inward flow of Qi, our body's connection to nature and the seasons.

Early Chinese doctors found that within the human body, meridians function in pairs, with one being relatively Yin and the other relatively Yang. This is reflected in organ pairs throughout the body. Thus, the Stomach and Spleen work together, with the Stomach being more active/Yang while the Spleen is comparatively Yin. The Large Intestine and Lung meridians also work together, as do the Small Intestine and Heart, Gallbladder and Liver, Urinary Bladder and Kidneys—all Yang and Yin organs, respectively.

The flow of Qi within the body is inherently connected to the flow of Qi in Heaven and Earth. Therefore, internal fluctuations of Yin Yang energy move in synergy with natural changes in the environment according to the seasons. As the energy from the sun (or Heaven) increases as we enter into springtime, so the Yang energy on the left side of the body rises. Similarly, as we transition into the Yin season of autumn, Yin energy begins to rise, affecting channels on the right side of the body.

We also see this interconnected relationship reflected in daily cycles. Yang energy is at its peak from sunrise to noon. As stated, this rising energy relates to organs and pathways on the left side of the body. The presence of Yin and Yang also impacts our cycles of rest. It is beneficial for a person to go to sleep before 11:00 p.m., because this is when the sun is considered to be

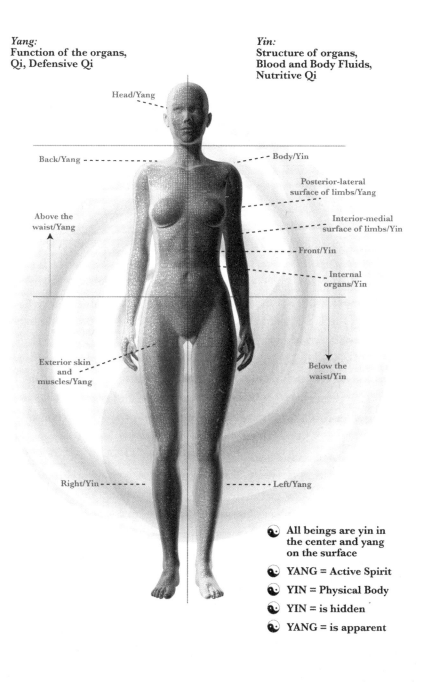

Yang:
Function of the organs, Qi, Defensive Qi

Yin:
Structure of organs, Blood and Body Fluids, Nutritive Qi

Head/Yang

Back/Yang

Body/Yin

Posterior-lateral surface of limbs/Yang

Above the waist/Yang

Interior-medial surface of limbs/Yin

Front/Yin

Internal organs/Yin

Exterior skin and muscles/Yang

Below the waist/Yin

Right/Yin

Left/Yang

- All beings are yin in the center and yang on the surface
- YANG = Active Spirit
- YIN = Physical Body
- YIN = is hidden
- YANG = is apparent

underneath the Earth, shifting away from the bright and active Yang energy, allowing Yin's restorative essence to penetrate.

During the day, the sun's energy travels through the Yin Earth, affecting channels on the right side of the body, thereby nourishing our inner Yin Essence. According to Chinese medicine, the Liver receives this Yin energy from the Earth within the time period of 11:00 p.m. and 1:00 a.m. That is why, to properly restore Yin, one should be asleep by this time. The state of sleep allows this Yin energy, or life-essence, to nourish the brain and spinal cord while penetrating deep into the organs systems of the body. Yin energy is essential for the health of vital organs, including the brain and spinal cord. During sleep, this energy helps to replenish and maintain the proper functioning of these organs.

Here is the fun part. As stated earlier, Yin and Yang are not absolute, but relative, concepts. For this reason, their associations within the body are fluid and interchangeable. For example, although the left side of the body is considered Yang, left pulse readings relating to the internal organs are Yin, as they reflect Blood and fluids within the body. The pulse readings on the left wrist correlate to the left kidney, which is also Yin in nature. Similarly, pulse readings on the right wrist connect to the right kidney, which is considered Yang as it relates to Qi and its transformation, production, and circulation throughout the body. The left kidney (Yin) is responsible for the cooling essence of the body, while the right kidney (Yang) is responsible for the heat required to transform and circulate Qi.

In practice, it is often useful to tap into the opposite energy for balancing Yin or Yang within the body. For example, if a practitioner is treating the Liver, which is located on the right side of the abdominal cavity, it is recommended they focus on acupoints on the left foot or lower leg, opposite the organ's location. By stimulating acupoints on the opposite side, practitioners aim to restore balance and harmony throughout the body. A proper balance of Yin Yang energies can help alleviate many issues rooted in an excess or deficiency of one of these two forces.

The Chinese classics view Yin organs as being more "precious" than the Yang organs of the body. This is because, while Yang is responsible for heat and the motive force underlying change and transformation, it is the nurturing quality of Yin that supports all life. It is characteristic of Yang to go to excess, to be bold, and to demand attention. By contrast, it is in the nature of Yin to become deficient, to withdraw, and to fail without fanfare. Therefore, supplying deficient Yin is generally more difficult than curbing excessive Yang. Thus, much of Chinese medicine and Qigong specifically target those precious Yin organs and their energy supply.

Massaging the Yang Organs

This exercise massages all Yang organs—which are, in essence, the entire digestive system. Thus, it is great for all digestive discomforts or complaints, both acute, such as nausea, and chronic problems, including constipation and heartburn. This exercise also aids in the daily development and replenishment of the postnatal Qi from the foods we eat.

1. Begin by standing in Wuji posture with feet shoulder-width apart, tailbone tucked, chin tucked (so as to raise the crown of the head), and the entire body relaxed and balanced.

2. Raise your arms in front of you to shoulder level while you inhale through the nose and into the lower abdomen. Keep the abdomen relaxed, and allow it to expand as it fills with air.

3. When you are ready to exhale, contract the abdomen, expelling the air as your arms swing back using about 70 percent power (that is, let inertia help carry them back).

4. Allow the arms to then swing up in front to continue the exercise.

5. Repeat these steps 50 times at first, gradually increasing to 150 times.

NOTES

1. Breathing should be natural so the swinging follows the breath in a regular, easy rhythm.

2. For acute problems, do this exercise as needed. For chronic issues, perform it once per day, ideally in the morning.

3. You can also do this exercise from a seated position (although standing is preferred).

Case History

A woman in her late fifties came in very upset because of pressure in her abdomen that was diagnosed by her physician as a prolapsed (fallen) uterus. Her doctor advised a hysterectomy. She also had fibroids, was prone to yeast infections, and reported that she bruised easily. I assessed the fundamental problem as a Qi deficiency disrupting the Spleen that, in turn, created a Yang deficiency that contributed to excessive dampness in the body. I recommended she radically change her diet by eliminating all cold and raw foods in addition to pasta, bread, and sugars (including fruit). I performed Curative Qigong to help warm and raise the uterus. After three sessions, her uterus returned to its normal position, and she has never gone back to her previous diet.

CHAPTER 5

THE VESSELS AND GATES

There are eight Extraordinary Meridians that help regulate the flow of energy through the body. They do this in two ways. First, they connect the main meridians. Their connections ensure that energy flows smoothly throughout the body and facilitates communication between the organs, supporting their proper functioning. Second, the Extraordinary Meridians serve as reservoirs of energy, which means they can supply deficiencies or absorb excesses in the main meridians. Because of this function, they are also called vessels. Two of the most important Extraordinary Meridians are the Governing and Conception Vessels. The Governing Vessel runs up the back of the body from the perineum up over the crown of the head and down the face to the cleft above the teeth, while the Conception Vessel runs up the front of the body from the perineum to the depression beneath the protrusion of the lower lip. (The perineum is the anatomical point between the sex glands and the anal sphincter.) Thus, together, these two meridians encircle the body on its vertical axis, both running very close to the surface. A third important Extraordinary Meridian is the Belt Vessel, which encircles the body at the waist. The path of these meridians also coincides with the network of the Central Nervous System, or CNS. Stimulating the CNS will fill the vessels and, by extension, all the meridians they supply.

Along these vessels, there are specific points where Qi—as well as Blood, other bodily fluids, and emotions—tend to get blocked. These points are known as "gates." There are seven gates of particular importance in Qigong practice:

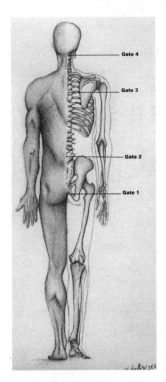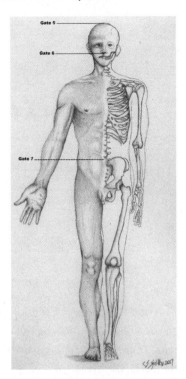

1st Gate: Perineum, or Hui Yin (Conception Vessel 1, or CV 1), located between the sex glands and the anal sphincter muscle.

2nd Gate: Gate of Life, or Ming Men (Governing Vessel 4, or GV 4), located on the spine exactly opposite the navel.

3rd Gate: Shen Dao, or Spirit Path (Governing Vessel 11, or GV 11), located between the shoulder blades.

4th Gate: Feng Fu, or Wind Mansion (Governing Vessel 16, or GV 16), located at the base of the skull.

5th Gate: Crown Point, or Bai Hui (Governing Vessel 20, or GV 20), located at the top of the head.

6th Gate: Mouth Point, or Shui Gou (Governing Vessel 26, or GV 26), located at the junction of the upper lip and the gums.

7th Gate: Sea of Qi, or Qi Hai (Conception Vessel 6, or CV 6), located about an inch and a half below the navel.

Stimulating and regulating the flow of energy in the vessels helps to regulate the flow of energy throughout the body in all of the Regular Meridians. The meditation known as the Microcosmic Orbit, or Jupiter Cycle, Meditation (also known as Small Heaven Breathing) specifically activates the Governing and Conception Vessels.

Microcosmic Orbit Meditation

The purpose of this meditation is to facilitate and reinforce the flow of Qi in the Conception and Governing Vessels. The first step is simply to become aware of the movement of the Qi; in later stages, you can develop power in guiding it. Ancient sages said that, with sincere practice, it will take one hundred days to fully open these two channels, or meridians. The time it takes is not important; even one day of practice will bring benefits!

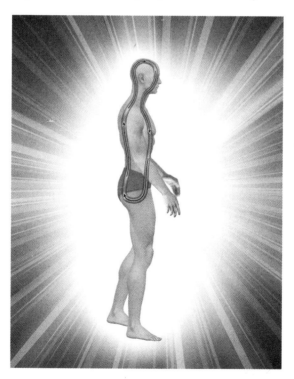

1. Start with the Three Regulations: steady breath, relaxed mind, Wuji posture (feet shoulder-width apart, shoulders relaxed and broad, tailbone tucked, Crown Point rising).

2. Place the tongue on the roof of the mouth behind the teeth. Lightly squeeze the anal sphincter muscle while relaxing the body.

3. As you inhale, guide Qi up the spine (up the Governing Vessel) to the crown of the head. If you cannot feel the Qi, you may imagine it as light, color, or blood and fluids moving upward.

4. As you exhale, guide the Qi from the Crown Point down the front of the face, entering the upper palate of the mouth to the point where the tongue touches the palate.

5. Continuing to exhale, guide the Qi down the front of the body (the Conception Vessel) to the perineum.

6. When the Qi reaches the perineum, repeat the exercise. Inhale, bringing Qi up the spine, then exhale bringing it over the crown of the head, down the face to the tip of the tongue and down the front to the perineum.

7. Repeat the exercise continuously. At the end, with your mind, bring the Qi to the lower Tan Tien and store it there.

NOTES

1. Initially, practice this meditation for 10 to 15 minutes per day.

2. At the beginning, while you may not feel the flow of Qi, use the length of one inhalation to visualize bringing it from the base of the spine to the crown of the head. Later, you can do it much faster, especially when you are aware of the sensation of Qi and its natural tendencies.

3. You may practice the Microcosmic Orbit Meditation in any position (standing, sitting, or lying down) and at any time. For example, you might do it while waiting, as when stopped at a traffic light or standing in line at a store; it can even be done while watching TV.

My Personal Experience

Although the ancient texts say it should take one hundred days, or about three months, to open the gates and feel the flow of Qi, for me it took six months. I did this meditation regularly, every day, and felt nothing . . . until one day I noticed the tip of my tongue pulsating, or vibrating, where it rested on the roof of my mouth. Since then, I have gradually been able to increase my awareness. At first, I could feel the Qi throughout its route in the Governing and Conception Vessels, then I could feel it in other organs. I believe doing the Microcosmic Orbit Meditation is a fundamental first step in following, and eventually directing, your Qi.

CHAPTER 6

FIVE ELEMENTS IN DETAIL

According to CCM and Curative Qigong®, the Five Elements arose from the observation of ancient sages that all phenomena in the universe stem from the movement of the five qualities: Fire, Earth, Metal, Water, and Wood. From the original void of Wuji arose Yin and Yang. Within this Wuji, Yin and Yang generated the Three Treasures: Heaven, Earth, and Man. This energy continues to unfold in the four divisions of Yin and Yang. These four divisions plus the Earth Element give us five phases of energy, commonly known as the Five Elements. The following is excerpted from *I Ching: The Book of Changes and the Unchanging Truth*, by Hua Ching Ni.

From the Five Elements come the "ten thousand things," or our material world. In Chinese medicine, Five Elements principles have had considerable influence on physiology, pathology, diagnosis, treatment and pharmacology. They have also been applied in the realms of Feng Shui and astrology.

Each of the Five Elements has specific characteristics and associations, as observed in nature over two millennia. Throughout this book, I will capitalize these five words when they refer to the Chinese concepts and not to physical objects. Thus:

> Fire has the traits of flaming upward, expansion, heat, dispersion, and dissipation.

> Earth is the sowing, reaping, and bringing forth of all phenomena. It carries the traits of harmony and balance and is essentially neutral.

> Metal is the working of change. It has the qualities of purification, refinement, elimination, reform, and gravity.

> Water has the traits of contraction, collection, and condensation.

> Wood has the characteristics of growth, initiation, release, and rejuvenation.

The Five Elements relate to each other in three cycles: the Creative Cycle, the Controlling Cycle, and the Destructive Cycle, as depicted in the figures below. In the Creative Cycle, one element is the "mother" of the other, giving it support to achieve harmony. In the Controlling Cycle, one helps to keep the other from growing out of control, maintaining harmony, while in the Destructive Cycle, one element will overact on another which can lead to disharmony.

Understanding these natural patterns of metamorphosis can help explain how organ systems affect one another and how to treat one system through another related one. They also help us understand how problems with one organ system can affect others. The meridians together with Five Elements principles describe and explain the interactions of the human body as a dynamic, holistic system.

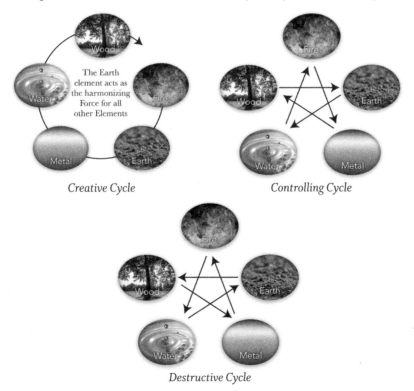

Creative Cycle   *Controlling Cycle*

Destructive Cycle

Collecting Heaven and Earth

The purpose of this exercise is to absorb Heavenly Yang and Earthly Yin energies, bringing them together in harmony. It is the opening practice for the five Organ Cleansing Exercises, which we will do next.

1. Start with the Three Regulations: steady breath, relaxed mind, Wuji posture (feet shoulder-width apart, shoulders relaxed and broad, tailbone tucked, Crown Point rising).

2. Spread the arms wide at shoulder level in a "T" position with palms facing up.

3. Raise the arms up over the head, palms facing each other.

4. As if rounding over a big ball, bend forward from the hips, keeping shoulders relaxed and the chin tucked toward the chest. Let the arms follow the movement.

5. When you have bent forward as far as you can, slowly drop the arms and hands toward the ground; let them dangle. Do not lock the knees; allow them to be loose.

6. Bend the knees as you curl up to a standing position, one vertebra at a time.

7. Repeat the exercise between 9 and 36 times (in multiples of 9).

Case History

I sometimes volunteer at elementary schools to teach kids about the different forms of Qigong and Tai Chi. After working with one class, the teacher later called to report what had happened on a museum field trip. On the way, kids were getting quite rowdy and out of control until one of the class leaders suggested, "Hey! Let's do that practice of Collecting Heaven and Earth that Mr. Shelton taught us!" So, the whole class started doing this exercise in the middle of downtown San Jose. The teacher reported that, as if by magic, all the kids calmed down and the rest of the trip went smoothly.

◈ CHAPTER 7 ◈

THE FIRE ELEMENT

Yin Organs:	Heart	Hours: 11 a.m. to 1:00 p.m.
	Pericardium	Hours: 7:00 to 9:00 p.m.
Yang Organs:	Small Intestine	Hours: 1:00 to 3:00 p.m.
	Triple Burner	Hours: 9:00 to 11:00 p.m.

Starting with this chapter, I will be discussing each of the Five Elements in terms of the meridians and organ systems with which they are associated. Because Yin organs are considered the most precious (for reasons mentioned in chapter 4), for each Element I will focus on its associated Yin organ. I will follow the Creative Cycle (as shown in fig. 12), starting with the Fire Element.

Finally, one more important note for all chapters that follow: Chinese references are not exactly the same as western labels for anatomical organs. For example, when CCM (Classical Chinese Medicine) refers to the Kidneys, it is referring to the energy of the Kidney system—not necessarily to the physical organs. Thus, if a Chinese medicine practitioner tells a patient that he/she has Kidney problems, it does not necessarily mean they have kidney disease. To remind the reader of this distinction, I will capitalize organ names when they refer to the Chinese concept and not when they refer to the physical organ.

The Fire Element has two pairs of meridians associated with it. One pair is the Heart and Small Intestine, the other is the Pericardium (the tissue surrounding the heart) and the Triple Burner. The Triple Burner is a conceptual energy system unique to CCM and Curative Qigong®. It has hours of activity, specific functions, points of access and control, etc., like other meridians, but it has no physical form.

In Chinese medicine, the Heart is said to rule the Blood and blood vessels. While the Liver is considered the Controller of Blood, the Heart is said to be the Governor. This means that the Liver allows Blood to move, while the Heart determines where the Blood needs to go. The Pericardium refers to the protective tissue of the heart. External pathogenic factors as well as emotions mostly attack the Pericardium before they affect the Heart.

The heart organ is located in the chest to the left. In CCM, it is believed that Heart energy is particularly important among all the organs as it controls the other viscera, including the bowels. The Heart has both Yin and Yang aspects. The Yin refers to the Blood controlled by the Heart and the Yang to the actual function, heat, and Qi of the Heart. The main functions of the Heart are: controlling blood circulation, taking charge of mental activities, and producing sweat as the fluid of the Heart. In terms of other body parts, the condition of the Heart is particularly expressed in the tongue, the sparkle of the eyes, and the complexion of the face.

Controlling Blood Circulation

Blood vessels are the tubes through which blood flows. They are linked to the heart, creating a closed system. CCM states that it is the Qi of the heart that keeps it beating and sending blood through the vessels. When Qi is sufficient, the heart can keep a normal rate and strength. The pulse of the heart reflects much about the Qi of the body and the condition of internal organs. Indeed, pulse diagnosis is an important form of assessment in CCM. You can think of assessing the pulse like assessing the flow of water in a hose. The condition of the hose—Is it flexible or stiff? Fully open or clogged?—as well as the power of the pump—Does it pump evenly or irregularly? Is it strong or weak?—will determine the quality and nature of the flow of water inside. A weak and empty pulse indicates a deficiency of Qi of the Heart, while a fine and weak pulse points to a deficiency of Blood of the Heart. A rough and rhythmical pulse reflects a decline of the Blood of the Heart.

In Charge of Mental Activities

The Fire Element rules the firing of the brain's neurons, synapses, and receptor sites. CCM asserts that nervous activities, like thinking, depend on the function of the Heart. When the functions of the Heart are normal, a person will have healthy levels of consciousness and mental activities. Abnormalities, like bipolar conditions, may be brought on by an insufficiency of Blood. Treatment for such kinds of mental problems is determined through analysis of the Heart condition.

Sweat Is the Extension of Blood

Bodily fluid is the fundamental component of blood and sweat. CCM states that profuse sweating indicates the Heart is using a lot of blood and Qi, which may result in palpitations and intense beating. Too much sweating depletes Yin and injures the Yang of the Heart. Those who have a lack of Yin in the Heart are likely to sweat at night. At the same time, sweating does not always indicate Heart problems. In CCM, no condition can be diagnosed from just one symptom.

Relationship with the Tongue and Face

CCM asserts that the condition of the Heart is expressed on the tongue and in the complexion of the face. With its many blood vessels, the face readily reveals the condition of the Heart. A rosy face, pink tongue, and sparkling eyes show that the Heart is functioning well and the person's spirit is strong. A white face and pale tongue suggest the Heart is not functioning well. Stagnation of Heart energy can be seen in a bluish face and a tongue that is dark purple or has a red tip.

On the psychological level, the Heart is also responsible for a person's appropriate interactions in time and place. In that sense, it allows for manners and propriety. On the emotional level, balanced Heart energy is expressed as the positive virtues of love and compassion; out of balance, it is expressed as over-excitation and frantic activity.

Fire Element Imbalance

Physical Signs:

- ☯ Lackluster eyes
- ☯ Heart palpitations
- ☯ Mental illness (bipolar, manic)
- ☯ Low or high blood pressure, dizziness

Emotional Signs:

- ☯ Anxiety with situations and people
- ☯ Forgetfulness
- ☯ Sense of vulnerability, jumpiness, chattiness
- ☯ Shyness
- ☯ Hysteria

Heart Meridian

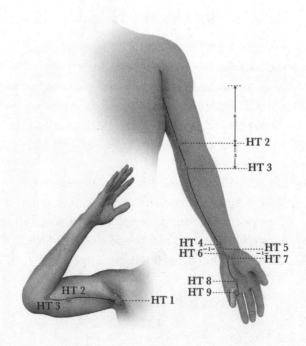

The Path of the Heart Meridian

The Heart meridian has three branches, each beginning in the heart. Two of the branches are internal; one runs through the diaphragm and connects to the small intestine, while a second branch runs upward along the side of the throat to the eyes. The third, external branch, runs across the chest from the heart to the lungs then descends and emerges in the underarm. On the surface of the body, it begins at the front crease of the armpit, runs down the inside of the arm, across the wrist and palm, and terminates at the inside tip of the little finger where it connects with the Small Intestine meridian.

USEFUL ACUPOINT ON THE HEART MERIDIAN

HT 9: This point is located at the tip of the pinky finger on the inner edge of the fingernail. Holding or massaging this point will normalize one's heart rate. Thus, whenever you feel your heart rate rise—for physical causes, such as a vigorous workout, or for emotional causes, such as stage fright and anxiety—hold your pinky and breathe deeply. You may also say the Heart sound, "HAAA," for extra help in restoring a normal heart rate.

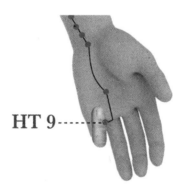

HT 9

Heart Cleansing Exercise

This exercise clears and harmonizes the energy of the Heart. It is useful for addressing any of the physical and emotional complaints listed above. You may use it for chronic conditions or acute situations, or you may use it simply to keep your Heart energy flowing smoothly.

THE MOVEMENT

1. Start with the Three Regulations: steady breath, relaxed mind, Wuji posture (feet shoulder-width apart, shoulders relaxed and broad, tailbone tucked, Crown Point rising). The tongue should be lightly touching the roof of the mouth behind the upper teeth.

2. Pull Down the Heavens three times.

3. Place the hands in front of the body, as if holding a small beach ball, at the height of the lower abdomen. The right arm should be horizontal (on top of the imaginary ball), palm down, parallel to the left arm below with the left palm facing up.

4. Turn your upper torso to the left. As you turn, your left arm rises and the forearm rotates to press the palm outward (fingers horizontal) while, at the same time, the right arm pushes to the left, under the left arm, palm facing out with fingers vertical. (In martial arts, this is a classic "block and punch" type of move.)

5. When you've reached a comfortable extension, allow the arms to come back to the starting position, but this time with the left hand on top, palm down, facing the right, palm up.

6. Next, mirror Step 3 on the right side. That is, turn your torso to the right. As you turn, raise your right arm, rotating the palm outward as the left arm pushes under it to the right, palm facing outward.

7. Return to center and repeat, left and right, at an even and gentle pace, between 3 and 36 times.

8. Close by Pulling Down the Heavens three times.

NOTES

1. To increase the efficacy of the exercise, you may say the Heart sound, "HAAA," while exhaling.

2. Breathing is a key aspect here. Be sure to inhale as you come to center; exhale as you turn and push out.

Case History

A middle-aged man who had had several heart attacks was working out at the gym. Because of his previous history, he was required to wear a heart monitor. During one session, his heart rate shot up to 180 beats per minute (BPM). His trainer, a client of mine, grabbed the man's pinky fingers and squeezed. Within a minute, the man's heart rate returned to a more normal level of 80.

CHAPTER 8

THE EARTH ELEMENT

| Yin Organ: | Spleen | Hours: 9:00 to 11:00 a.m. |
| Yang Organ: | Stomach | Hours: 7:00 to 9:00 a.m. |

The Spleen, according to Chinese medicine, is different from the anatomical organ as described in western medicine. CCM states that the Spleen is located in the middle of the body cavity and is the main organ of digestion. Its Yin aspect is the material structure while its Yang aspect is the function. The Spleen's function, which is absolutely fundamental to the health of the body, is transforming food essence and liquid into Blood. The Spleen is also responsible for containing organs in their proper places, such as the blood in its vessels and uterus and anus in their respective positions. The Spleen has a relationship to the muscles, limbs, and lips.

Transporting, Distributing, and Transforming Nutrients

CCM states that, after going through the stomach, food essence enters the Spleen where it is separated into what is useful and what is not. The waste then travels through the pylorus to the small intestine. What is not waste is said to "rise" to the Lungs where it is combined with air and sent to the Heart to produce Blood. If the Spleen is not functioning properly, a person may suffer from lack of appetite, indigestion, fullness, distension in the epigastrium (the upper middle section of the abdomen—see image below), loose stools, lassitude, and/or loss of weight, among other symptoms. The Spleen is also said to absorb and transport water. If the Spleen does not absorb water properly, the body will retain water, resulting in edema, dampness, and/or diarrhea. Thus, the Spleen absorbs both food essence and water at the same time, and both functions are connected. An abnormal functioning of one will lead to the abnormal functioning of the other.

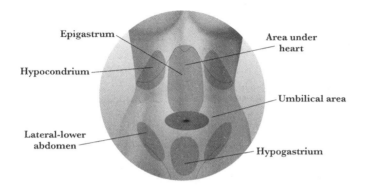

Keeping Blood Circulating Within the Vessels

The Spleen keeps blood circulating normally within the vessels. If there is a lack of Qi, blood will not flow normally and will escape from the vessels. When this happens, it can result in such symptoms as blood in the stool, uterine bleeding, or spontaneous nosebleeds.

On a broader, energetic level, the Earth element transforms food essence into the textures and activities of human life and is responsible for creative change in life. The Spleen, in particular, acts as the harmonizing force between all other organs. The Earth Element is also associated with being centered in thought and action. Spleen energy, when in balance, is expressed as the positive virtues of serenity, calmness, and centeredness. Out of balance, it is expressed as worry, over-intellectualizing, and excessive thinking. Conversely, anxiety and mental stress can cause problems in the Spleen and, from there, the entire digestive system. Naturally sweet and bland foods nurture the Spleen.

Earth Element Imbalance

Physical Signs:

- ☯ Loose stools

- ☯ Anemia

- ☯ Major depressive disorders

- ☯ Obsessive compulsive disorder (OCD)

- ☯ Allergies

- ☯ Underweight or overweight

- ☯ Diabetes

- ☯ Prolapse of any organ (e.g., uterus)

- ☯ Craving for sweet or starchy foods (carbohydrates)

Emotional Signs:

- ☯ Apathy

- ☯ Brooding

- ☯ Over-intellectualizing or overthinking, prolonged worry or anxiety

The Path of the Spleen Meridian

The Spleen meridian originates at the outside corner of the big toe. It then runs along the inside of the foot, turning in front of the inner ankle bone. From there, it ascends straight up the lower leg behind the shinbone, up the inner aspect of the knee and thigh into the abdominal cavity. It runs internally to the Spleen and connects with the Stomach. The main branch continues on the surface of the abdomen, running upward to the chest, where it again penetrates internally to follow the throat up to the root of the tongue, under which it spreads its Qi and Blood. An internal branch leaves the Stomach, passes upward through the diaphragm, and enters the Heart, where it connects with the Heart meridian.

Spleen Meridian

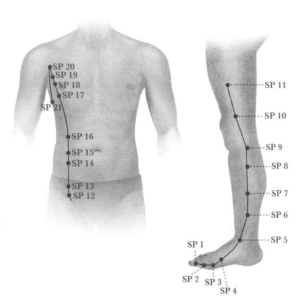

USEFUL ACUPOINTS ON THE SPLEEN MERIDIAN

SP 6: This point is located on the inside of the ankle, three fingers' width above the ankle bone. Massage this for digestive problems, excess phlegm or mucus in the chest, and also for arthritic pain (which represents an accumulation of phlegm in the joints). Three Yin organ meridians converge at this point, so it is particularly valuable for restoring balance in all Yin functions. This point can also be used to build or tonify Blood.

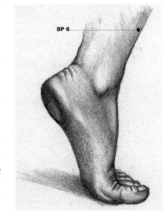

SP 21: This point is located under the armpit, more or less directly in the center. Massage this area to relieve emotional aspects of Spleen imbalance, such as worry or brooding. This point connects directly with the Spleen, so it is particularly potent.

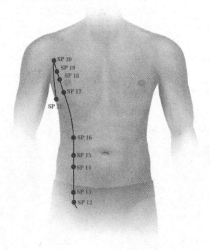

Spleen Cleansing Exercise

This exercise clears and harmonizes the energy of the Spleen. On the physical level, it helps restore good digestive functioning. On the emotional level, it calms the mind. Practicing this movement can help reduce anxiety and worry while re-establishing one's central stability. It is especially recommended for people who spend a lot of time feeling worried or stressed, and for those who simply think too much.

THE MOVEMENT

1. Start with the Three Regulations: steady breath, relaxed mind, Wuji posture (feet shoulder-width apart, shoulders relaxed, tail-bone tucked, Crown Point rising). The tongue should be pointing down behind the lower teeth.

2. Pull Down the Heavens three times.

3. Bring the hands together in front of the body, just above the head, with the tips of thumbs and index fingers together, forming the shape of a diamond.

4. Gaze upward through this diamond.

5. Continue to gaze through the diamond while twisting the torso to the left, back to center, then to the right. Repeat at a slow, deliberate, and steady pace. Your hands should rotate around the center of the diamond, and your knees should remain more or less facing forward. The main point is to compress and release your abdominal cavity, where the Stomach and Spleen are.

6. Repeat the exercise 3, 9, or 36 times.

7. Close by Pulling Down the Heavens three times.

NOTES

1. To increase the efficacy of the exercise, you may say the Spleen sound while gazing through the diamond. The Spleen sound is: "HUUU" (hhh-ooo).

2. Remember to breathe deeply into your lower Tan Tien.

3. The easiest way to keep the diamond still is to find something on the ceiling, or above you, that falls in the center of the diamond. Then, as you twist, make sure that point of focus remains in the center of the diamond.

4. The most common error with this exercise is failing to keep the shoulders relaxed. Feel the weight of your shoulder blades, and allow them to simply fall.

Case History

Parents brought in their 5-year-old son because he was having chronic nosebleeds. Doctors had recommended cauterizing the blood vessels. After talking to the boy, I learned he was very anxious about the prospect of starting kindergarten. Stress depletes Spleen energy; sugar was no doubt also involved, another stress on the Spleen. I recommended a change of diet, eliminating sugar and processed foods. I taught him the Spleen Cleansing Movement and suggested that, whenever he felt anxious, he should say the Spleen sound. The treatment worked, and the problem was resolved.

CHAPTER 9

THE METAL ELEMENT

Yin Organ:	Lung	Hours: 3:00 to 5:00 a.m.
Yang Organ:	Large Intestine	Hours: 5:00 to 7:00 a.m.

The Metal Element relates not only to the respiratory system, but also to the immune system (including the lymphatic system), large intestine (colon), and the skin. The Metal Element is said to control Wei Qi, also called Defensive Qi. This particular type of Qi has a shielding effect and, thus, is considered analogous to our immune system.

Anatomically, the lungs are made up of two lobes located in the chest. They connect to the larynx, bronchi, and trachea, opening to the external environment through the nose. In Chinese medicine, the Lung is divided into the Yin of the Lung (the material structure) and the Qi of the Lung (the functions of the lung); the term "Yang of the Lung" is rarely used. The Yang organ paired with the Lung is the Large Intestine. The functions of both are expressed in the quality of the skin and strength of the voice.

The Lungs are involved in regulating the interaction between the body and air in three ways: through inhalation and exhalation, by opening and closing the pores of the skin, and by producing and maintaining Defensive Qi. Because purified Qi of inhaled air is involved in the production of Blood, the Lungs are, therefore, also involved in nutrition. During inhalation, water is sent to the Kidneys, so Lung function also affects fluid balance in the body.

Purifying Inhaled Air

The most important, and perhaps most apparent, function of the Lungs is to extract clean Qi from inhaled air. This purified essence of the air is combined with food essence from the Spleen and sent to the Heart where it becomes Blood.

Producing Defensive Qi

The Lungs produce the very important Wei Qi, or Defensive Qi, which is the body's first line of defense against pathogens from the environment. Wei Qi is closely related to the health of the skin and water metabolism (see below), particularly the opening and closing of the skin's pores. When Defensive Qi is weak, the body easily succumbs to attack from external pathogens, such as parasites and infectious diseases.

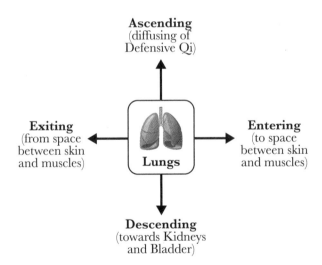

Activating the Flow of Qi Downward

Because the Lungs are the uppermost Yin organ of the body, their Qi must descend. When it does not descend, such symptoms as coughing, asthmatic breathing, and stuffiness in the chest can occur. It can also cause shortness of breath, tiredness, and drowsiness.

Maintaining Normal Water Metabolism

When the Lungs are functioning properly, inhalation will send water downward to the Kidneys and Urinary Bladder. Failure of the water supply to these organs can result in dysuria (the inability to urinate), edema (swelling), and/or phlegm-retention conditions.

The Lungs are also responsible for supplying the skin and hair with the bodily fluid they need to stay moist and bright. By spreading Qi between the muscles and skin, the Lungs regulate the opening and closing of the skin's pores and keep the muscles warm. As part of the immune system, healthy skin defends the body from outside pathogenic factors. Unhealthy skin is associated with symptoms such as profuse sweating and vulnerability to the common cold.

Metal Element Imbalance

Physical Signs:

- Shoulders rolled forward

- Phlegm

- Chronic coughing

- Dry skin (eczema)

- Stools dry and hard, or loose

- Aversion to cold or heat

- Susceptibility to colds or flu

Emotional Signs:

- Lack of willpower

- Disinclination to talk

- Lack of assertiveness

- Feelings of sadness, disappointment, or despair

- Hypersensitivity

☯ Feeling exposed or vulnerable

☯ Inability to attain one's goals

The Path of the Lung Meridian

This meridian starts at the region of the Stomach, moves down to connect with the Large Intestine, then rises back up through the diaphragm to the Lungs. It continues up to the middle of each side of the collarbone then out each arm, passing in front of the bicep muscle to the center area of the elbow crease. It then travels through the wrist to the thumb pad, finishing at the outer side of the base of the thumbnail.

Lung Meridian

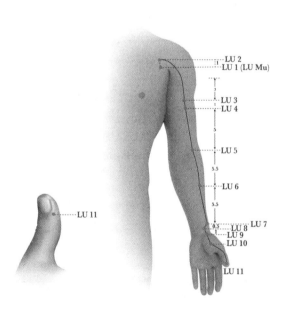

USEFUL ACUPOINTS ON THE LUNG MERIDIAN

LU 1 & 2: These two points are very close to each other underneath the clavicle in the crease where the shoulder and the chest meet (if you move your shoulder forward). When you have phlegm or a cough that produces phlegm, vigorously massage these points to warm them up.

LU 7, 8 & 9: These points are located at the wrist crease on the radial artery. Rubbing or massaging the three points can help reduce a fever and/or subdue a cough, especially in children. For a more thorough stimulation of the Lung meridian, starting at the wrist crease, vigorously rub the inside of the arm from the wrist to about 2 inches above the wrist toward the elbow.

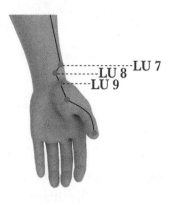

Lung Cleansing Exercise

This exercise clears and harmonizes the energy of the Lungs. It is useful for reducing any of the physical or emotional complaints listed above, and it may also be used as a general health practice. It is particularly beneficial during the autumn to help strengthen the Lungs. It can also help release excess sadness and sorrow.

THE MOVEMENT

1. Start with the Three Regulations: steady breath, relaxed mind, Wuji posture (feet shoulder-width apart, shoulders relaxed and broad, tailbone tucked, Crown Point rising). The tongue should be resting gently between the upper and lower teeth.

2. Pull Down the Heavens three times.

3. With eyes gazing forward, allow the arms to float up in front of the body to shoulder height, palms facing down.

4. While inhaling, spread the arms out to the side, palms down, as though opening curtains; this movement expands the chest.

5. Turn your palms up and, while exhaling, bring your arms back to the front and center of your body, closing your chest.

6. Repeat in a continuous flowing motion.

7. End by Pulling Down the Heavens three times.

NOTES

1. It is recommended to do this 3 to 6 times for health maintenance, or 9 to 36 times (in multiples of 9) when addressing a particular problem.

2. You may enhance the efficacy of this exercise by saying the Lung sound, "SSSS," while exhaling.

Case History

A two-year-old had several seizures, which were terrifying for the parents. Their western physician predicted that after a child has one seizure, he is likely to have more by age five or six and offered no preventive measures. The parents refused to accept this prognosis, believing something could be done. They took the infant to an acupuncturist who prescribed an herbal formula to improve digestion. He also taught the parents to open the baby's arms in the Lung Movement and advised them to rub the wrists and arms along the Lung meridian. The parents reported that the baby never had another seizure.

· CHAPTER 10 ·

THE WATER ELEMENT

| Yin Organ: | Kidneys | Hours: 5:00 to 7:00 p.m. |
| Yang Organ: | Urinary Bladder | Hours: 3:00 to 5:00 p.m. |

The Water Element relates to the Kidneys and the Urinary Bladder. It controls the skeletal system (bones), reproductive system (including the testes and ovaries), and the endocrine system (which includes the adrenals, pancreas, hypothalamus, thyroid, pituitary gland, pineal gland, and thymus). Thus, the Kidneys rule the overall constitution, health, and longevity. The health of the Kidneys is considered the foundation for the balance of all other internal organs. The Yin aspect of the Kidneys is storing the Essence of Life (Jing) and water; the Yang aspect is serving as the "Life Gate of Fire," the motive force for transformation in the body. Because of these fundamental functions, the Kidneys are affected by any chronic disease.

The Kidneys rule the bones and, therefore, the production of bone marrow; the teeth are considered a surplus of the bones. The Kidneys open into the ears and the hair on the head. Ancient texts state that when the ears and Kidneys are harmonized, one can hear five tones. The moistness and vitality of the hair on the head are related to Kidney Essence. (The hair also depends on Blood for nourishment, which is why the hair on the head is also referred to as a surplus of Blood.)

Kidney Functions

The main functions of the Kidneys are: storing the Essence of Life, regulating water metabolism, and controlling and promoting inhalation.

STORING THE ESSENCE OF LIFE

There are two components of the Essence of Life. The first is the Prenatal Essence of Life, or Prenatal Qi. Although given at conception, it can be somewhat strengthened through food and nutrition and is capable of being transformed into the Qi of the Kidney. Kidney Qi contributes to the growth, development, and replacement of the body, for example, the production of teeth. The body grows as Kidney Qi increases. When the body reaches puberty, the Qi of the Kidney is at its peak. It then initiates the production of sperm in boys, eggs and menstruation in girls. As the body ages, Kidney Qi weakens, diminishing reproductive capabilities.

The second component of the Essence of Life is acquired, Postnatal, Qi. It is derived only from food. The Spleen and Stomach transform food essence into Postnatal Qi, which is then transported to the five viscera and six bowels. When there is insufficient Postnatal Qi for the body to function, the Kidneys will supply it from the reservoir; conversely, when there is a surplus, the Kidneys will store it. So, when any organ is not functioning correctly, the Kidneys need to be nourished, because Kidney Qi will be relied upon to supply any deficiencies.

The Kidneys' Essence of Life aids in making bone marrow, which nourishes the bones. When the Kidneys are functioning well, bones and teeth are strong. Conversely, when they are weak, both the bones and teeth will lack nourishment as well. The Essence of Life also turns into Blood, which nourishes the hair. When the Kidneys are functioning well, the hair will be strong and shiny. Withered hair and premature hair loss or graying can be a sign of weak Kidneys. Finally, the Kidneys also influence brain function. When Kidney Qi is strong, thinking and memory will be sharp and clear.

REGULATING WATER METABOLISM

The Kidneys maintain fluid balance in the body. Bodily fluids are responsible for transporting nutrients to organs and tissues and for carrying waste out of the tissues. The Kidneys play an important role in both functions by either releasing excess or retaining needed water. When the Kidneys are functioning well, urination will be normal. When not properly functioning, the Kidneys may release too much, causing issues like polyuria (excessive urination) and frequent urination. When the Kidneys do not release enough urine, it can lead to oliguria (scant urination) and edema (swelling and excess accumulation of water in body tissues).

CONTROLLING AND PROMOTING RESPIRATION

According to Chinese medicine, the Kidneys aid in inhalation and the Lungs in exhalation. When the Kidneys are not functioning well, inhaling will be difficult, which can result in dyspnea (difficult or labored breathing) and severe panting.

Kidney Dysfunctions

According to CCM and Curative Qigong®, Kidney Essence is like a battery charge that powers your life. You can never have too much, but you can use it up. This is why all Kidney disease patterns involve a deficiency of some sort. Sources of potential deficiencies—that is, ways your Kidney Essence can become exhausted—fall into six categories: hereditary, emotional, sexual, chronic illness, aging, and overwork.

HEREDITARY WEAKNESS

Prenatal Qi, or Life Essence, is formed at conception. Its quality is determined by the condition of each parent's Essence, Heavenly Qi, and the environment at the time of conception. If the parents' Essences are weak, meaning they had weak constitutions at conception, the child can also be weak and may have such symptoms as poor bone development and teeth, enuresis (inability to hold urine), thin or weak hair, and, in extreme cases, cognitive disabilities. Since a person's vital energy naturally declines with age, conceiving late in life can also weaken the constitution of the child. When Prenatal Qi is weak, the person must pay particular attention to other factors in order to avoid a stress or drain on this irreplaceable vital force.

EMOTIONS

Fear, fright, shock, and anxiety make Qi descend, especially in children. It can happen to anyone; a traumatic experience, or something you witness can cause shock, depleting your Kidney Qi. In adults, such a depletion may be the root cause of insomnia and mental restlessness.

SEXUAL ACTIVITY

Excessive orgasms weaken the Kidneys, because they are directly related to Kidney Essence; this also includes masturbation. The Heart and Kidneys are closely related and, during orgasm, one may often experience heart palpitations. Conversely, Heart deficiency caused by sadness and anxiety can weaken the Kidneys and cause impotence or a lack of sex drive, as well as coldness in the limbs and enuresis (involuntary urination).

CHRONIC ILLNESS

Any long-lasting, chronic condition will create a deficiency of Kidney Yang and/or Kidney Yin.

AGING

Kidney Essence naturally declines with age. In fact, in Chinese medicine, the process of aging is defined as the manifestation of a decrease in Kidney Essence. Hence, as a person ages, they experience a decline in all functions controlled by Kidney Essence, namely hearing, bone density, sexual function, memory, and hair.

OVERWORK

This means mental and physical work for long periods of time or burning the candle at both ends. In modern society, this is the most common cause of depleted Kidney Yin. Long work hours (particularly mental work) in unhealthy environments, emotional stress, lack of relaxation and exercise, improper and irregular meals, poor sleep, etc. draw directly on Yang energy. When the Yang energy normally used for these functions is exhausted, the body starts using up Yin Essence. Because Yin Essence is generally harder to restore, its depletion leads to problems that are more difficult to treat. In all of these cases, eliminating the drain on Yang Essence is the first step to recovery.

Water Element Imbalance

Physical Signs:

- Arthritis
- Poor memory
- Ringing of the ears
- Bone degeneration

- Premature hair loss and/ or graying
- Involuntary loss of semen
- Lack of sex drive
- Infertility
- Shortness of breath
- Hearing loss
- Inadequate or excessive urination

Emotional Signs:

- Lack of motivation and drive, apathy
- Being fearful or apprehensive
- Inability to confront issues
- Inertia

The Path of the Kidney Meridian

The Kidney meridian begins underneath the base of the small toe, moves over to the center of the foot at the base of the ball of the foot, then runs across the sole, emerging along the arch. It makes a circle below the inner ankle, then ascends along the inside of the lower leg, behind the Liver and Spleen meridians, to the inner knee crease. It continues on the inside of the thigh, then enters the torso near the base of the spine. One branch connects internally with the Kidneys and Urinary Bladder. From there, it emerges on the surface of the abdomen above the pubic bone and runs upward over the abdomen and chest, ending at the collar bone. Another internal branch ascends to connect with the Liver, Lungs, and Heart, terminating at the base of the tongue.

Kidney Meridian

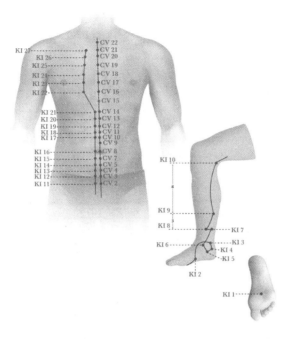

USEFUL ACUPOINTS ON THE KIDNEY MERIDIAN

KI 1: This point is known as the Bubbling Spring point. It is located in the center of the ball of the foot. Pat it with a cupped hand for insomnia due to an overactive mind. It is also good to rub to relieve shock. Or, to relieve a cold, rub liniment oil on the point before bed.

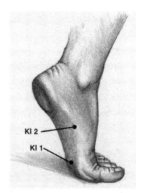

KI 2: This point is located on the inner side, or instep, of the foot where the bulge of the big toe starts. Massage this point to tonify the body or to relieve aching feet. It may also be used for problems of the reproductive system, such as infertility or nocturnal emissions.

Kidney Cleansing Exercise

This exercise clears and harmonizes the energy of the Kidneys. Use it to relieve any of the physical or emotional symptoms listed above, or as part of a general health routine.

THE MOVEMENT

1. Start with the Three Regulations: steady breath, relaxed mind, Wuji posture (feet shoulder-width apart, shoulders relaxed and broad, tailbone tucked, Crown Point rising).

2. Pull Down the Heavens three times.

3. Roll the tip of the tongue back to the soft palate on the roof of the mouth.

4. Place the back of the left hand on the lower back, over the region of the right kidney.

5. Bring the right arm up to the left side of the body, about eye level and parallel to the floor, with the palm facing outward.

6. Inhale as you sweep your arm to the right, gazing at the back of the right hand.

7. Exhale as you lower the right hand and bend forward at the waist, scooping down and across with your right arm in front of your body, from right to left.

8. Continue this in a circular motion. That is, inhale as you sweep your arm at eye level to the right, then exhale as you scoop/sweep your arm to the left at knee level.

9. Repeat several times, then begin on the left side.

10. Finish by Pulling Down the Heavens three times.

NOTES

1. As part of a daily health routine, perform the exercise three times on each side. When targeting a specific problem, repeat 9 to 36 times (in multiples of 9) on each side.

2. To increase the efficacy of the exercise, you may say the Kidney sound, "FUUU" (fff-ooo), when exhaling.

3. The left kidney represents Kidney Yin, which is the foundation of the cooling essence of the body, including sweat, blood, and bodily fluids, while the right kidney represents Kidney Yang, the motive force for heat and transformation in the body. Thus, it is important to do both sides equally.

Case History

A client had a flu bug that had lasted for eight months; we call this a "febrile disease," as it involved a low-grade fever in the body. Her western physician had not been able to help her recover. She saw a Chinese doctor who prescribed herbs and performed acupuncture. This cured the flu, but she then developed a chronic case of vertigo (Meniere's Disease). Again, the western physician couldn't help. When she came to me, I assessed the problem as a depletion of Kidney Essence. I gave her moxa (a warming treatment), acupressure, and Qi projection on specific Kidney points. Her homework was to do the Kidney movement daily, particularly whenever she had an incidence of vertigo. Within a week, she saw improvement, and within 4 to 6 weeks, her symptoms were gone.

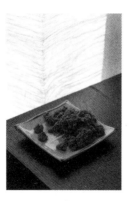 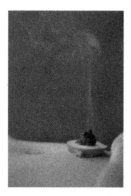

CHAPTER 11

THE WOOD ELEMENT

Yin Organ:	Liver	Hours: 1:00 to 3:00 a.m.
Yang Organ:	Gallbladder	Hours: 11:00 p.m. to 1:00 a.m.

In the Chinese system, the Wood Element corresponds to the Liver and Gall-bladder energies in the human body. Anatomically, the liver organ is located in the upper right part of the abdomen, behind the lower part of the rib cage. In Chinese medicine, the main functions of the Liver concern filtering, storing, and regulating Blood and Qi. The quality of Liver energy is specifically reflected in the quality of the tendons, ligaments, sinews, nails, and eyes.

In Chinese medicine, the Liver is often compared to trees, as both tend to "spread out freely." The Liver's main function is to spread Qi throughout the body. It accomplishes this in three ways: regulating mind and mood, promoting digestion and absorption, and keeping Qi and Blood moving normally. In Chinese medicine, the Heart and Liver regulate the flow of vital energy and Blood, which results in an even temper, feelings of happiness, and relaxation. But when the Liver does not function well, it will result in anxiety, irritability, anger, and resentment. Modern society places a particularly heavy stress on the Liver, both in the type of food we eat and the stresses inherent in daily life. Road rage is a typical example of Liver Qi imbalance, seen through the lens of Chinese medicine.

The Liver's function of regulating the flow of energy in the body aids the Spleen in distributing nutrients and water, therefore contributing to good digestion. An unhealthy Liver can affect the Spleen in a negative way, resulting in poor appetite, belching, vomiting, and diarrhea.

The Liver's function of regulating the flow of energy directly affects the flow of Blood. Erratic Blood flow can result in symptoms throughout the lower abdomen, particularly in women, affecting the menstrual blood.

Wood Element Imbalance

Physical Signs:

- Floaters or blurred vision
- Eye or facial tremors
- Unsettled sleep, waking between 1:00 and 3:00 a.m.
- Menstrual irregularities, especially blocked or reduced flow
- Hypochondria pain (i.e., pain just below the ribs)
- Chemical sensitivities
- Food allergies
- Hives or red, painful skin eruptions
- Uneven energy throughout the day
- Migraine headaches
- Constipation
- Nausea

Emotional Signs:

- Depression
- Sudden outbursts or feelings of overwhelming rage and anger
- Inability to handle stressful situations

The Path of the Liver Meridian

The Liver meridian begins at the pinky side of the big toenail. It then goes over the top of the foot in front of the inner ankle, along the inner side of the shin bone, and up past the knee. It continues up the inner side of the thigh to the pubic region where it encircles the genitalia before entering the lower abdomen and ascending to the Liver and Gallbladder. It then spreads across the diaphragm and ribs, ascends to the neck, throat, and eye system, and ends at the top of the head.

Liver Meridian

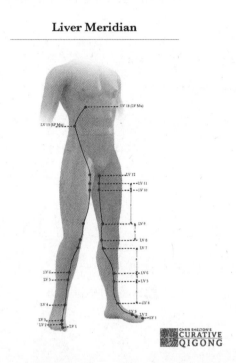

USEFUL ACUPOINTS ON THE LIVER MERIDIAN

LV 3: This point is located on the top of the foot between the tendons leading to the big toe and the next toe. It can be used to drain excess energy from the Liver channel; if it is painful when touched, massage will help any symptom resulting from excess Liver energy. Use this for acute attacks of anger, or massage regularly for harmonizing menstrual irregularities, disturbed sleep, eye problems, etc.

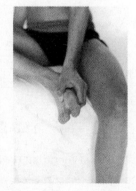

LV 13: This point is located on the top of the floating ribs on both sides of the body, directly down from the armpit. Massage this point when you have

a "stitch" in your side, for depression, or to help control the functions of the Gallbladder and Spleen.

LV 14: This point is located below each nipple in the spaces between the ribs. It connects directly with the Liver, and massaging it can help reduce intense feelings of anger or resentment. (This is a point that is tender to the touch for most people.)

Front Mu Points

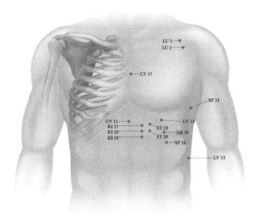

Liver Cleansing Exercise

This exercise clears and harmonizes the energy of the Liver. It is useful for reducing any of the physical or emotional complaints listed above. On an emotional level, it targets and reduces the negative emotions of anger and frustration, while encouraging kindness and compassion.

THE MOVEMENT

1. Start with the Three Regulations: steady breath, relaxed mind, Wuji posture (feet shoulder-width apart, shoulders relaxed and broad, tailbone tucked, Crown Point rising). The tongue should be pointing straight up, touching the roof of the mouth.

2. Pull Down the Heavens three times.

3. Bring the right hand, palm up, to the right side of the body. Position it at the ribs.

4. Stretch the left hand forward, wrist flexed so the palm faces out, as if you are trying to push something away from the body.

5. Pull the left arm/palm back as you push the right arm/palm out. The left palm pulls in to the left side of the ribs, facing up, while the right arm extends forward, palm vertical, facing away from you. In other words, the left hand goes back to where the right hand started and the right hand pushes out as the left did. Widen the eyes and stretch the tendons of the fingers on your outstretched hand.

6. Repeat this exchange. There should be a rolling effect of the palms as they pass one another midway through the movement.

7. Finish by Pulling Down the Heavens three times.

NOTES

1. Do this daily to keep Liver energy flowing smoothly, but particularly if you have issues with anger, resentment, or frustration.

2. Keep your shoulders relaxed.

3. To increase the effect of the exercise, you may say the sound for the Liver, which is "SHUU" (shh-ooo).

Case History

A woman, who appeared to be very fit and was a fitness trainer, came in with back problems. Reading her face, I saw signs of unresolved anger, which I suspected involved deep-seated regrets. She denied this, saying she had dealt with those issues, and believed that a healthy diet and exercise were enough to maintain good health. Even so, I suggested she have a cardiovascular checkup. Reports showed that both carotid arteries were 76 percent blocked. She's now practicing the Yin organ exercises and sounds, with particular emphasis on those for the Liver and Heart. At the same time, she is working on her emotional health, spending time to become aware of and resolve issues. She says she now realizes that emotions, as well as diet and exercise, are a critical component of overall health.

CHAPTER 12

RESTORING EARTH'S ENERGY

According to Chinese Medicine, the practice of Restoring Earth's Energy relates to your Post-Heaven Essence and is associated with the Earth Element. As such, it connects to the energy of the Stomach and Spleen.

Pre-Heaven Essence is related to your Kidneys and is gathered at the time of conception between your parents, the environment, and God. This essence determines how well one is able to recover from stressful situations and establishes the underlying energy a person has to ward off disease and increase the quality of life. It predetermines how long your life will be, and as you age, naturally becomes reduced. Increased stress, burning the candle at both ends, and toxins taken into the body will increase the rate at which the Pre-Heaven Essence declines.

One of the ways to keep this life-essence from diminishing so quickly is by observing what you put into your stomach, relating to Post-Heaven Essence that can be cultivated through proper diet and a healthy lifestyle. This means being aware and selective of the type of food you eat and eating according to your element type and the seasons.

Our Stomach Qi naturally begins to decline at age 45, for both men and women. Therefore, it is important to pay attention to the above recommendations as well as to remain mindful while eating. Don't stand or walk when you eat. Chew your food deliberately and slowly. While eating, don't engage in intense conversations or arguments, and avoid watching TV.

Make sure to avoid ice-cold drinks! Drinking ice water or cold drinks interferes with the process of digesting food, as it causes your blood vessels to shrink. This can slow down the process of digestion and cause food to be digested improperly, which can lead to nutrients being lost or not absorbed by the body. Consequently, you can catch a cold or other illness more easily, because this decreases the proper functioning of the immune system, in which the Stomach and Spleen play a key role. These things occur because coldness injures the Spleen, creating excess mucus in the body. Furthermore, drinking cold water also slows the function of the Heart. This is because, according to Chinese medicine principles, cold substances impede the smooth flow of blood circulation due to their contracting effect on the body.

The Stomach and Spleen are most active between 7:00 and 11:00 a.m.; therefore, your largest meal of the day should be at this time. This is the time of day when Yang energy is rising. It is also the time of day when you will be able to derive the most nutrients from the food you eat.

In the following Qigong practice, we are mindfully gathering Earth energy while pulling the breath and Qi into the Middle Burner, a region you will learn more about in chapter 18. This helps to restore balance and harmony within the Stomach and Spleen, slowing down the aging process and balancing the other internal organs.

The practice below is meant to restore health to the digestive system. The Stomach and Spleen are considered the Qi thoroughfare for which the body's energy is collected and spread throughout to sustain life. As discussed before, the Stomach and Spleen are connected to our Post-Heaven Essence that is nourished by the food and drink we put into our bodies. Emotionally, nourishment comes from kind words or actions directed toward others and, in turn, the kind words or actions we receive.

According to Classical Chinese medicine, the mouth and lips are connected directly to the Stomach and Spleen. So, having proper nourishment comes not only from the food we eat but also the words we say and what others say to us. Therefore, words can either enhance our body and mind, or they can cause harm to both. Mentally, the Spleen is harmed by over-intellectualizing and brooding, as well as by the negative emotions of worry and anxiety. Other aspects often taken for granted that harm the Spleen and Stomach include how you eat; watching TV or arguing while eating, eating while standing up, eating too late, or eating foods that are contraindicated for your constitution will also damage the proper functioning of both.

The importance of the essence being properly derived from food and drink is that it gives energy back to the Pre-Heaven Essence residing in the Kidneys that determines how long your life will be. Therefore, being emotionally balanced and nurturing both the Pre-Heaven and Post-Heaven Essences through proper diet and healthy eating practices will enhance your ability to age gracefully.

The Practice

1. Begin this meditation from a standing Wuji posture, with the sacrum tucked and feet shoulder-width apart, shoulders relaxed and broad, Crown Point rising.

2. With the breath long, steady, even, and deep into the lower Tan Tien, begin to settle your mind.

3. Pull Down the Heavens three times and relax the body.

4. Inhale, reaching your arms up toward the sky. As you exhale, make soft fists with the hands, rolling the arms in toward the chest with palms facing inward.

5. Continuing to exhale, slightly bend the knees while folding at the waist, and pull the fists into your midsection at the end of the rib cage on the xiphoid process.

6. As you pull into the midsection, imagine a golden light filling up into the Stomach and Spleen. At the same time, make the "HUUU" (hhh-ooo) sound under your breath.

7. Repeat the practice.

8. Do this practice between 9 and 36 times (in multiples of 9).

9. Finish by Pulling Down the Heavens three times and storing the energy back into the lower Tan Tien, one inch below the naval.

CHAPTER 13

THE HEART HEALING SOUND

The next six practices are some of my favorite Qigong healing exercises. Called the Six Healing Sounds, the first is connected to the Heart and is also referred to as Dry Cry.

In earlier chapters, we performed movements that benefit the five internal organs of the body. For example, the Heart Cleansing Exercise helps to sedate, or tonify, emotions of the Heart as well as physical imbalances of the organ itself.

We are now going to dive deeper by incorporating the actual sound vibrations associated with each organ. When giving public talks, I leave the audience with three major takeaways. The first is conscious breath, the second, Shaking the Tree (which I really love), and the third is the Heart Healing Sound, or Dry Cry.

With all healing sounds, we are emphasizing the sound vibration associated with various organs. The corresponding colors and emotions that harm organs sometimes get stuck; these practices allow for a gentle release.

The Heart Healing Sound is something we already do all the time without realizing it. For example, if you have lost a loved one or pet, or had a recent break up, your body will automatically sigh as a way to release the painful emotion that's trapped in the Heart. Or, after a laughing attack, the first thing the body naturally does is make the "HAAA" sound, or sigh, and the reason it does this is because you have temporarily created an imbalance in the Heart, and the body's intelligence is attempting to readjust and regain balance.

According to Classical Chinese medicine, the Heart is the emperor or empress of the body and dictates how much of an emotion will be expressed or suppressed. It is disturbed by such negative emotions as: over-excitation, excess joy (or lack thereof), mania, abandonment, and loneliness. But because of its proximity to the Lungs and the Lungs' correlation to grief and sorrow, the Heart is also easily affected by the feelings of sadness and loss.

What's so cool about these practices (besides being something your body instinctively does whenever you have an emotional stress) is that you can do them vocally as well as underneath your breath. You can also practice them in public; this means you don't have to suppress emotions as they arise, which creates inflammation and, eventually, disease. Instead, you'll be able to let go of the negative emotion as it arises, or as you feel it. It's a very simple and effective practice.

Because you can practice each sound audibly or in audibly, if you're in public and something upsets you, pronouncing the sound underneath your breath will allow you to release the energy before it becomes stored in the body and organs. Between the two options, speaking the sound audibly will create a stronger vibration, yet both are powerful. If you are someone who has suffered a severe loss and have a "stuck" feeling in the pit of your throat (like you swallowed a plum seed) this is the Qi of grief or sorrow that is trapped in the area and can be released by this practice. So, if you've experienced an upset and suddenly have this stuck feeling in your throat, as you practice the Heart Healing Sound, you will want to lift the chin and imagine the circumstance leaving from the throat as a dark cloud, going several feet away from the body, down deep into the ground.

The Heart is considered the most important of all internal organs. It helps in the transformation of food Qi into Blood and is responsible for the circulation of blood throughout the body. In Classical Chinese medicine, the Lungs, Spleen, and Liver also play a crucial role in blood circulation.

The Heart and Blood help determine the strength of an individual's constitution, though connected to the essence of the Kidneys. When the Heart is strong, circulation is good; a person will have a full figure and a robust constitution. Since the Heart governs Blood, blood vessels, and distribution of blood throughout the body, the state of the Heart can therefore be reflected in one's complexion. If Heart Qi is strong, the complexion will be rosy and lustrous.

Our Heart houses the Mind, also called Shen, or spirit. This represents the complex mental faculties of the mind which are closely linked to the

Heart. The Shen indicates the whole sphere of mental, emotional, and spiritual aspects of a human being, but it also encompasses the mental, emotional, and spiritual phenomena of all internal organs, particularly the Yin organs.

If the Heart is subjected to prolonged or trapped emotional traumas, it will show up as numerous health conditions that we don't normally associate with the heart itself. For example, unresolved feelings of abandonment and loss can create a deficiency of Blood in the Heart. When Heart Blood is weak or deficient, a person will have a poor constitution and a lack of internal strength; the complexion will be pale or bright white. If Blood becomes stagnant, the complexion will turn bluish-purple. When there is an excess of heat present in the Blood, the complexion will be red, and the mind will suffer. One will experience diminished mental activity in memory, thinking, and consciousness, along with disturbed sleep. Numerous conditions that directly affect the heart will manifest, like atrial fibrillation, high/low blood pressure, anxiety, depression, heart palpitations, and angina (chest pain).

The amazing thing about this simple and easy-to-do practice is that, when done regularly along with proper diet, sleep, exercise, and hydration, you can help avoid or alleviate the above conditions. More importantly, you will have a tool to cope with the various emotions that attack the Heart and may otherwise show up as disease over time.

The Practice

1. Do this practice from a seated, standing or lying down position.

2. If seated or standing, start off in Wuji posture.

3. Focus on the breath spreading into the Heart center as you inhale. While pulling the breath deep into your Heart, imagine a pink or red cloud filling the space within and around it.

4. Now focus on an event, past or present, that has created an emotional disturbance felt in your Heart. (This may be any of the full range of emotions.)

5. As you focus on the event, bring it into the present moment as much as possible. Who and what was involved? Were there any smells or colors associated with the situation? Feel it now as though it has just happened. Once you have this connection established,

visualize the pink cloud filling up into the Heart center as you inhale. As you exhale, make the "HAAA" sound, and imagine that circumstance leaving (from either your throat or mouth) like a dark cloud, going several feet away from the body and deep into the ground.

6. Do this over and over.

7. As you inhale, focus on bringing in the positive virtue of the Heart, which is love.

8. Try doing a few of the repetitions audibly, then inaudibly under the breath.

9. Again, if at any point you're feeling emotions that cause your heart rate to increase or trigger pain in the area of the heart, practicing the sound immediately will release the negative energy and keep it from becoming stored in the body.

10. To finish the practice, Pull Down the Heavens three times and store the energy in the lower Tan Tien.

PHYSICAL SIGNS OF FIRE IMBALANCE:

- Shortness of breath

- Forgetfulness

- Insomnia

- Heart palpitations

- Angina

- Myocardial infarction

- Mental illness

- Sudden blackouts

- Atrial fibrillation

- Dizziness

EMOTIONAL SIGNS OF FIRE IMBALANCE:

- Anxiety (with situations and people)

- Shyness

- Sense of vulnerability or wanting to withdraw

- Feeling jumpy or chatty

- Hysteria

- Mental confusion

CHAPTER 14

THE SPLEEN HEALING SOUND

This practice benefits the Spleen and Stomach as well as the pancreas. In particular, it is used to harmonize the Spleen and cleanse it of the negative emotional components of worry, brooding, obsessive thinking, and anxiety. When done properly, this practice helps bring forth the positive virtues of the Spleen: centeredness, serenity, and peace of mind.

The Spleen is the main organ responsible for the transportation and transformation of food essence. Essentially, the Spleen controls the process of transforming the essence of food into Qi and sending it up to the chest to be made into Blood. The Spleen is ruled by the Earth Element which allows food to become the essence and activities of human life. It is also responsible for fueling creative change in one's life. The Spleen and Stomach are considered part of a person's Postnatal Qi because of their anatomical locations in the visceral cavity. The Spleen acts as the harmonizing force between all other organs and is associated with a grounded centeredness in thought and actions. Spleen energy manifests in the lips and opens into the mouth, controlling saliva, the bodily fluid it is associated with.

The Spleen houses the Intellect (Yi), meaning when the Spleen is functioning properly, one can reason and understand objectively. Spleen Qi influences our capacity for thinking, studying, concentrating, focusing, and memorizing. Though other organ systems, like the Heart and Kidneys, also play a role in thinking, it is said that when the Spleen functions properly, we can concentrate and commit information to memory more easily. On the flip side, studying or engaging in mental work that requires extended periods of concentration will create a deficiency of Spleen energy.

In addition, if negative emotions associated with the Spleen are not thoroughly processed, illness will manifest as a result of the imbalance. A deficient Spleen caused from excessive worry will inhibit a person's mental capacities. They may become stubborn and unable to understand things objectively. Conditions like cysts, cancer, fibroids, prolapses, blood disorders, excessive phlegm, chronic bloody noses, and weak muscles may arise. As a result of the deficiency, a person may then crave sugar and carbs, further exacerbating the above conditions and creating issues with weight gain.

The Practice

1. Do this practice from a seated, standing, or lying down position.

2. If seated or standing, start off in Wuji posture.

3. Focus on the breath filling up into the Spleen (located on the left side of the abdomen) as you inhale.

4. While pulling the breath deep into the Spleen, imagine a yellow or orange cloud filling the space in and around the organ.

5. Now focus on an event, past or present, that creates a sense of worry or anxiety for you.

6. As you focus on the event, bring it into the present moment as much as possible. Who or what was involved? Were there any smells or colors associated with the situation? Feel it now as though it has just happened.

7. Once you have this connection established, visualize the yellow/orange cloud filling up into your Spleen as you inhale. As you exhale, make the "HUUU" (hhh-ooo) sound.

8. Imagine that circumstance leaving from your mouth like a dark cloud, going several feet away from the body and deep into the ground.

9. Do this over and over.

10. As you inhale, focus on bringing in the positive virtues of the Spleen: peace of mind and a feeling of centeredness.

11. Try doing a few of the sounds audibly, then inaudibly under the breath.

12. Again, if at any point in time you experience emotions that cause you anxiety or if you catch yourself overthinking, practicing the sound immediately will release the negative energy and keep it from becoming stored in the body.

13. To finish the practice, Pull Down the Heavens three times and store the energy in the lower Tan Tien.

PHYSICAL SIGNS OF EARTH IMBALANCE:

- Pain in the joints
- Loose stools
- Gastritis
- Hemorrhoids
- Anemia
- Obsessive compulsive disorder (OCD)
- Dragging of feet while walking
- Allergies
- Being underweight or overweight
- Diabetes
- Edema
- Prolapsed uterus
- Craving sweet or fatty foods

EMOTIONAL SIGNS OF EARTH IMBALANCE:

- Lack of motivation
- Boredom
- Lack of excitement
- Despondency
- Stubbornness
- Over-intellectualizing (overthinking)
- Constant worry or anxiety
- Avoidance of activities once considered enjoyable

▪ CHAPTER 15 ▪

THE LUNG HEALING SOUND

This practice works with the Lungs and Large Intestine. The negative emotions that attack the Lungs are those of sadness, grief, disappointment, shame, and guilt. The positive virtue that comes forth once the grief and sadness is processed properly is courage.

As discussed in chapter 9, the Lungs are ruled by the Metal element. They have many functions outside of respiration and are considered the most superficial organ of the body via their connection to the nose and the role they play in controlling the opening and closing of pores on the skin. When a person effectively processes the negative emotions of the Lungs, the immune system will be robust, the voice full, and the skin supple and moist. They will have good circulation and the Blood will be strong.

Most people understand what grief and disappointment are. At the same time, it's important to differentiate between the emotions of shame and guilt. Guilt is when we feel like we have done something "bad" or wrong. Shame is the deep (though false) belief that we are unworthy, flawed, or otherwise unlovable for the thing we did or the way we are. It causes us to retreat, to pull away from others, to poison our self-talk, and to act in ways that perpetuate the experience of being an unworthy person. Shame tells us we're never good enough, and it asks us, "Just who do you think you are?" It tells us we're intrinsically "bad" and undeserving of love, or that if people really knew us intimately, they would reject us. This inadvertently affects our health and, in particular, the soul that is stored in the Lungs, called the Corporeal Soul (Po).

The Corporeal Soul is the aspect of consciousness that resides in the body and returns to the Earth after death. It is affected by all emotions, especially disappointment, grief, shame, guilt, and sadness. These emotions are associated with and stem from the inability to process loss in all forms, manifesting as repressed grief and sorrow.

This part of the soul is also known as the "animal" soul. It controls our primal instincts and can be seen in the body's basic physiological functioning. However, it can also be seen as concerning our physical and material needs, as in the process of collecting and holding onto what is needed to survive. This is discernment, where instinct and judgment occur within and concerning the surrounding world. Another trait of the animal soul is the ability to experience emotion and pain without dwelling upon events.

When the Corporeal Soul is out of balance due to grief, disappointment, shame, and guilt, conditions like asthma, low energy, Blood deficiencies, skin disorders, inertia, weak constitution, and breathlessness arise. The amazing thing about the Lung healing sound is that, when done properly, a person will experience greater vitality while strengthening the immune system.

The Practice

1. Do this practice from a seated, standing, or lying down position.

2. If seated or standing, start off in Wuji posture.

3. Focus on the breath filling up into your Lungs as you inhale.

4. While pulling the breath deep into the Lungs, imagine a white or silver cloud filling the space within and around them.

5. Now focus on an event, past or present, that creates feelings of grief, sadness, loss, disappointment, shame, or guilt within you.

6. As you focus on the event, bring it into the present moment as much as possible. Who or what was involved? Were there any smells or colors associated with the situation? Feel it now as though it has just happened.

7. Once you establish this connection, visualize the white/silver cloud filling up into your Lungs as you inhale. As you exhale, make the "SSSS" sound, like the sound of air being let out of a tire.

8. Imagine that circumstance leaving from your mouth like a dark cloud, going several feet away from the body and deep into the ground.

9. Do this over and over.

10. As you inhale, focus on bringing in the positive virtue of the Lungs: courage.

11. Try doing a few of the sounds audibly, then inaudibly under the breath.

12. Again, if at any point in time you experience emotions that cause you to feel sadness, grief, etc., practicing the sound immediately will release the negative energy and keep it from becoming stored in the body.

13. To finish the practice, Pull Down the Heavens three times and store the energy in the lower Tan Tien.

PHYSICAL SIGNS OF METAL IMBALANCE:

- Shoulders rolled forward
- Phlegm containing blood
- Chronic coughing
- Edema
- Vulnerability to colds or flu
- Dry skin (eczema)
- Dry hair
- Either dry, hard or loose stools
- Aversion to wind

EMOTIONAL SIGNS OF METAL IMBALANCE:

- ☯ Lack of willpower
- ☯ Dislike of talking
- ☯ Lack of assertiveness
- ☯ Feeling sadness or disappointment
- ☯ Feeling exposed
- ☯ Inability to attain one's goals
- ☯ Hypersensitivity
- ☯ Feeling of despair

CHAPTER 16

THE KIDNEY HEALING SOUND

This practice works to balance the Kidneys and Urinary Bladder. The negative emotions that affect the Kidneys are fear and shock. When we look at shock, we take into account all the various ways it affects the body. Shock includes surviving a severe illness or traumatic accident, as well as burning the candle at both ends. It also includes witnessing something tragic and experiencing other traumatic events like war, physical or mental abuse, and neglect. The Kidneys are ruled by the Water element. The positive virtues that come forth when in balance are gentleness and willpower.

Willpower (Zhi) is the soul that manifests in the Kidneys. The meaning of the soul, as used here, represents the immaterial, emotional, and intellectual aspects of a human being and shows up as action orientation, depending upon its function. There are two aspects of willpower, the Yang and the Yin. The Yang aspect of willpower in the Kidneys inspires one to make decisive efforts and fundamental commitments, allowing an individual to take responsibility for their life. The Yin aspect of willpower recognizes desire and the unfolding of life. It is based on intention and does not require much work. Yin willpower is about the direction we move toward that can only be seen or noticed once we look back and realize our total development over time. It is about fate, destiny, the unknown, and death.

When the Kidneys are strong, willpower will be strong. The mind will be focused on goals that it sets for itself, and it will pursue them in a single-minded way. When we are affected by fear, shock, or burning the candle at both ends for too many years, it will create weakness in the Kidneys. When the Kidneys are weak, willpower will be lacking, and the mind will be easily discouraged and swayed from its aims. Lack of willpower and motivation are often key aspects of mental depression, and because the Kidneys are the root of our Prenatal Essence, many other diseases listed below can show up as well. For more information on Kidney function, please refer to chapter 10. A main benefit of practicing the Kidney Healing Sound is that you will find you have greater focus and a lot more energy.

The Practice

1. Do this practice from a seated, standing, or lying down position.

2. If seated or standing, start off in Wuji posture.

3. Focus on the breath filling up into your Kidneys as you inhale.

4. While taking a long, deep breath into your low back, imagine a blue or black cloud filling each kidney on either side of the spine, just below the ribs.

5. Now focus on an event, past or present, that creates fear, or any shocking, traumatic situation you have witnessed or experienced.

6. As you focus on the event, bring it into the present moment as much as possible. Who or what was involved? Were there any smells or colors associated with the situation? Feel it now as though it has just happened.

7. Once you establish this connection, visualize the blue/black cloud filling up into the Kidneys as you inhale. As you exhale, make the "FUUU" (fff-ooo) sound.

8. Imagine the circumstance leaving from your mouth like a dark cloud, going several feet away from the body and deep into the ground.

9. Do this over and over.

10. As you inhale, bring in the positive virtues of the Kidneys: gentleness, wisdom, and willpower.

11. Try doing a few of the sounds audibly, then inaudibly under the breath.

12. Again, if at any point in time you experience a situation that causes you to feel fearful, or if you've come out of a shocking or terrifying situation, practicing the sound immediately will release the negative energy and keep it from becoming stored in the body.

13. To finish the practice, Pull Down the Heavens three times and store the energy in the lower Tan Tien.

PHYSICAL SIGNS OF WATER IMBALANCE:

- Arthritis
- Poor memory
- Ringing of the ears
- Infertility
- Bone degeneration
- Premature hair loss and/or graying
- Involuntary loss of semen
- Lack of sex drive
- Infertility
- Shortness of breath
- Hearing loss
- Dizziness
- Tiredness
- Frequent urination

EMOTIONAL SIGNS OF WATER IMBALANCE:

- Lack of motivation and drive

- Being fearful or apprehensive

- Lack of motivation to live or get out of bed

- Inability to confront issues

- Inertia

CHAPTER 17

THE LIVER HEALING SOUND

This sound balances the organ systems of the Liver and Gallbladder. The negative emotions that affect the Liver and Gallbladder are those of anger, old anger, frustration, hatred, irritation, and being too controlling. The positive virtues that come forth when these dissipate are kindness and creativity.

The Liver is ruled by the Wood element and houses the Ethereal Soul (Hun) which resides in the body and returns to Heaven after death. When anger, old anger, and resentment are held onto for too long or are not processed properly, it will affect the functioning of the Ethereal Soul, creating physical and emotional dysfunctions. The Ethereal Soul is Yang in nature (as opposed to the Yin Corporeal Soul) and, after death, transcends the body to flow back into a world of subtle, non-material energies.

The Ethereal Soul is said to influence the capacity to plan ahead and find a sense of direction in life. A lack of direction in life or mental confusion can be compared to the wandering of the soul, alone in space and time. Thus, if the Liver (in particular Liver Blood) is flourishing, the Ethereal Soul will be firmly rooted and can help us to plan out our lives with wisdom and clear vision. If, however, Liver Blood is weak, it will not be rooted and cannot provide a sense of direction in life. If Liver Blood or Liver Yin is very weak, at times, the Ethereal Soul may even leave the body temporarily during sleep or just before falling asleep. Those who suffer from severe Yin deficiency may experience a sensation as though they are floating in the moments just before falling asleep; this is said to be due to a "floating" Ethereal Soul not rooted in Blood and Yin.

The Ethereal Soul is also the source of life dreams, vision, aims, projects, inspiration, creativity, and ideas. It is described as the coming and going of the Mind (Shen). This means it gives the mind the necessary and vital dimensions of life (i.e., the components listed above). Without these, the mind will become sterile and a person will suffer from depression. On the other hand, the Mind needs to restrain, somewhat, the coming and going of the Ethereal Soul to keep it under check. It also needs to integrate, in an orderly fashion, all of the ideas spurting forth from the Ethereal Soul into our psyche. It is like an ocean of ideas, dreams, projects, and inspirations, and the Mind can cope with only one at a time. If the Ethereal Soul brings forth too much material from its ocean without enough control and integration by the Mind, a person's behavior will become somewhat chaotic and, in extreme cases, positively manic. Practicing the Liver Healing Sound gives us the tools necessary to better process anger and resentment and turn them into the positive virtue of being kind and gentle to others as well as ourselves. It allows for creative expression and the fulfillment of dreams. For more information on the function of the Liver, please refer to chapter 11.

The Practice

1. Do this practice from a seated, standing, or lying down position.

2. If seated or standing, start off in Wuji posture.

3. Focus on the breath filling up into your Liver, on the right side of the abdomen, as you inhale.

4. While pulling the breath deep into the Liver, imagine a green cloud filling the space within and around it.

5. Now focus on an event, past or present, that creates feelings of anger, rage, or resentment, or bring to mind areas in life where you are too controlling.

6. As you focus on the event, bring it into the present moment as much as possible. Who or what was involved? Were there any smells or colors associated with the situation? Feel it now as though it has just happened.

7. Once you establish this connection, visualize the green cloud filling up into the Liver as you inhale. As you exhale, make the "SHUU" (shh-ooo) sound.

8. Imagine the circumstance leaving from your mouth like a dark cloud, going several feet away from the body and deep into the ground.

9. Do this over and over.

10. As you inhale, bring in the positive virtues of the Liver: gentleness and creativity.

11. Try doing a few of the sounds audibly, then inaudibly under the breath.

12. Again, if at any point in time you experience a situation that causes you to feel anger or resentment, practicing the sound immediately (and underneath your breath if you have to) will release the negative energy and keep it from becoming stored in the body.

13. To finish the practice, Pull Down the Heavens three times and store the energy in the lower Tan Tien.

PHYSICAL SIGNS OF WOOD IMBALANCES:

- Dizziness
- Floaters or blurred vision
- Numbness of the extremities
- Dry nails
- Unsettled sleep
- Acid reflux
- Hypochondriac pain
- Ringing in the ears
- Chemical sensitivities
- Menstrual block or reduction in flow

- Sexual dysfunction

- Eye or facial tremors

- Convulsions

- Uneven energy throughout the day

- Migraine headaches

- Constipation

- Nausea

EMOTIONAL SIGNS OF WOOD IMBALANCE:

- Feeling depressed

- Sudden outbursts of anger

- Feeling overwhelming rage and anger

- Inability to handle stressful situations

- Disturbed sleep

CHAPTER 18

THE TRIPLE BURNER
HEALING SOUND

The Triple Burner is one of the most elusive topics in Chinese medicine and has sparked controversy for centuries. Chinese doctors have especially debated whether the Triple Burner has a "form" and if it is an actual organ or simply a "function" of the body.

The literal Chinese translation for this word means "three that burn." The Triple Burner (San Jiao) is considered the sixth of the Yang organs. It is the source for the functional relationship between all other organ systems, mainly the Lungs, Spleen, Liver, Small and Large Intestines, Urinary Bladder, and Kidneys. It is said that it is the pathway that links the internal organs yet has no distinct shape or form. The Upper Burner has been described as "a mist," corresponding to the idea that the vaporized water in the Lungs is later spread throughout the body. The Middle Burner is said to resemble "a foam," referring to the digestive actions of the Stomach and Spleen, while the Lower Burner is known as "a drainage ditch" due to its role in ridding the body of waste.

The Upper Burner is housed in the head and chest area, and includes the Heart and Lungs. The Middle Burner is located below the chest and above the navel, controlling the Spleen and Stomach, and the Lower Burner connects with the abdominal region of the Liver, Gallbladder, Intestines, Urinary

Bladder, and Kidneys. As a whole, the Triple Burner is responsible for the transformation, transportation, and excretion of fluids. It is like a system of canals that channels water through the proper regions and then out of the body. This ensures that fluids are transformed, transported, and excreted properly. The mechanism allows the Upper Burner to control bodily fluids, as in sweat between the skin and the muscles. The Middle Burner then aids in fluids produced by the Stomach that provide moisture to the body and integrate Blood. The Lower Burner primarily governs urine and the fluids absorbed by the small intestine.

Its function is like other Yang organs. That is, to receive food and drink, digest and transform it, then transport it in for nourishment and out for the excretion of waste.

The mental and emotional aspects of the Triple Burner are determined by its dual nature as it pertains both to the characteristics of Fire (Heart) and Wood (Liver). The Triple Burner relates to Fire exteriorly and gets pulled into the Pericardium, but is also connected to Original Qi and the Gate of Fire (Ming Mien). As a result, the Triple Burner plays a crucial role in assisting the Mind and Ethereal Soul, especially while forming personal relationships. When functioning properly, it allows for an appropriate balance between outgoing energy directed toward others and giving back equally to ourselves. The Triple Burner influences the Liver in promoting a free flow of emotions that are then expressed and, therefore, not repressed and held within the body. Just as the Triple Burner controls the movement of Qi within all organs and structures, it also provides a smooth flow of Qi between the Mind and Ethereal Soul so emotions do not turn into depression or moodiness. The following practice is easy to do and is great for harmonizing all of the internal organs and their associated emotions and functions.

Triple Burner

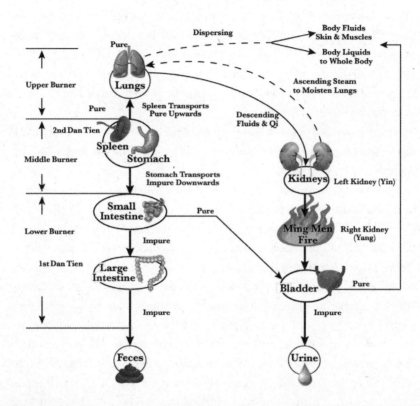

The Practice

1. Start from a seated, standing, or lying down position.

2. If seated or standing, come into Wuji posture.

3. Focus on the breath filling your entire chest and abdominal cavity.

4. As you inhale, gather the energy and air around you by cupping your hands, reaching your arms out wide to the sides and pulling the Qi toward your chest or eyebrows/third eye.

5. Upon exhalation, make the sound of "ZZZZ" while moving your hands down, palms facing the body, fingers pointed toward the ground.

6. Guide the sound throughout your body and allow the breath to flow along with your hands as they move from the chest down into the lower abdomen. (As you exhale, guiding the breath and vibration down into the lower abdomen, you will notice the sound will change pitch from a higher to a deeper tone.)

7. Inhale again, gathering the energy and air in front of you by drawing your arms in toward your chest, making the "ZZZZ" sound. However, this time, as you exhale and allow the sound to vibrate while the hands move down onto the lower organs and belly, imagine a red cloud clearing out each of the three Burners.

8. If any emotions or feelings come up, acknowledge them and allow them to disperse deep into the ground several feet away from the body as you exhale.

9. Do this 9 to 36 times (in multiples of 9).

10. Try a few repetitions of the "ZZZZ" sound audibly, then inaudibly under the breath.

11. Finish the practice by Pulling Down the Heavens three times, and store the energy in the lower Tan Tien.

PHYSICAL SIGNS OF TRIPLE BURNER IMBALANCES:

- Externally contracted diseases
- Febrile diseases
- Invasion of Wind Cold or Wind Heat
- Gastrointestinal problems
- Insufficiency of Blood

EMOTIONAL SIGNS OF TRIPLE BURNER IMBALANCES:

- Easily agitated
- Mental confusion
- Hysteria
- Despondency
- Explosive temper
- Reclusive
- Depression
- Anxiety disorders
- Obsessive Compulsive Disorder (OCD)
- Bipolar conditions
- Mania

CHAPTER 19

OPENING THE THREE TAN TIENS

The following is excerpted from *Chinese Medical Qigong Therapy: A Comprehensive Clinical Text*, by Jerry Alan Johnson.

According to Chinese physiology, the Three Tan Tiens are vital energy centers located in the center of the body along the Taiji Pole, also referred to as the Center Core of Light. They store energy much in the way a battery does. The Tan Tiens correspond to the seven chakras found in yoga, Hinduism and Ayurvedic practices. The Governing Vessel (GV) and Conception Vessel (CV) connect on the outside of the Taiji Pole by entering at the top of the head at GV 20 and exiting at CV 1 on the perineum. Each Tan Tien corresponds to the anatomical location that is the center of magnetic and electrical vibrational charge. When Qi moves through the body's Tan Tiens and through the Taiji Pole, energy is absorbed into the internal organs and surrounding tissues as well as internal/external meridians and collateral channels. Each Tan Tien acts like a reservoir, redistributing energy throughout the body and finally supplying it to the Defensive Qi (Wei Qi).

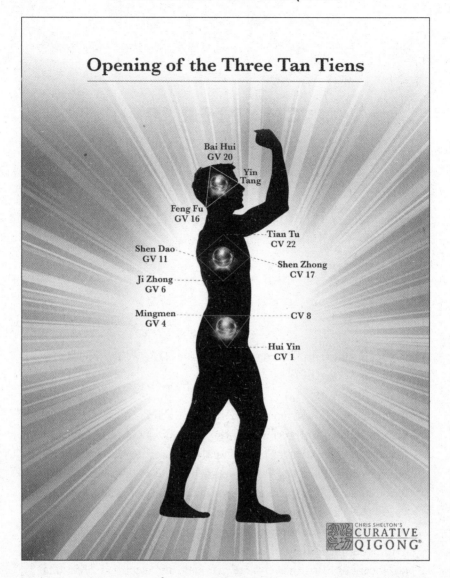

Opening of the Three Tan Tiens

Bai Hui
GV 20

Yin
Tang

Feng Fu
GV 16

Tian Tu
CV 22

Shen Dao
GV 11

Shen Zhong
CV 17

Ji Zhong
GV 6

Mingmen
GV 4

CV 8

Hui Yin
CV 1

CHRIS SHELTON'S
CURATIVE
QIGONG

Lower Tan Tien

This area is regarded as the storage of our physical strength. It is associated with the color blue. The triangular shape of the lower Tan Tien helps to draw Qi up from the Earth. It is here that the Earthly Yin energy is gathered through the three Yin channels of the legs: Liver, Kidney, and Spleen. As it enters the perineum, this energy is converted into heat which fuels our survival instincts. This heat in the lower Tan Tien is associated with physical energy and the Kidneys. With meditation practices focused on the lower Tan Tien, a person can transform water from the Kidneys and heat from the Ming Mien into a "mist" of Qi that circulates throughout the body.

The lower Tan Tien stores our Essence, or Jing Qi, as well as the Yin and Yang energies of the body. The Kidney Essence within this region circulates through the Eight Extraordinary Vessels, particularly the Governing, Conception, and Thrusting Vessels. Some practitioners believe the lower Tan Tien is located in the uterus in women and the prostate and seminal vesicle in men; however, the process of Qi transformation occurs in the ovaries and testicles. Thus, blockages in the lower Tan Tien often manifest as an inability to achieve orgasm, sexual dysfunction, organ prolapse, enuresis, edema, and bowel issues, to name a few.

While practicing Qigong, the Earth's energy is the first thing a practitioner connects with. This is because Yin energy from the Earth helps to balance out any excess Yang energy that may build up during Qigong practice. The correspondence between the lower Tan Tien and Earth energy relates to the grounding and stabilizing qualities associated with both. Earth is a grounding element, representing stability, nourishment, and rootedness. Similarly, the lower Tan Tien is a source of stability and strength within the body's energy system. By cultivating and strengthening the energy within the lower Tan Tien, one can enhance their connection to Earth energy.

The lower Tan Tien sends and receives kinetic impulses, records life experiences, and responds instinctively to emotion. When you have a gut feeling about something, the lower Tan Tien is responsible. The CV 1 and GV 4 points of the region represent the Yin and Yang of the lower Tan Tien and are necessary for cultivating inner power for internal martial arts (the cultivation of Qi), healing, and spiritual transcendence.

LOCATION OF THE LOWER TAN TIEN

The lowest point of the lower Tan Tien is in the perineum, between the sex glands and the anal sphincter muscle, Hui Yin (CV 1). The front point of the lower Tan Tien is located at CV 4, one inch below the navel, and the back at GV 4, Ming Mien. The sound to open the chambers of the lower Tan Tien is "HAREEM."

The Middle Tan Tien

The Heart is the primary organ related to the middle Tan Tien, the second being the Lungs, and the third, the thymus. The middle Tan Tien collects Qi and represents the body's energetic reservoir for mental and emotional vibration and energy. The middle Tan Tien is known as the Sea of Qi in the chest. It is comprised of Zong Qi (Ancestral Qi), Gathering Qi, and Essential Qi. Zong Qi and Yuan Qi (Prenatal Qi) work together to maintain healthy functioning of the Heart and Lungs by regulating water passageways, transforming food essence into Blood and Qi, strengthening the immune system, and regulating sweat and body temperature.

As you refine your Essence, the middle Tan Tien helps to transform fluid in the chest into a steam-like energy that is sent up to the upper Tan Tien, refining the spirit (Shen) in the Heart center. Because the Heart, in turn, houses the Mind and negative emotions of the Heart, it can easily become drained of necessary Qi. Practices aimed at cultivating and balancing the energy of the middle Tan Tien can, therefore, influence emotional well-being and mental clarity.

The middle Tan Tien connects with Defensive Qi (Wei Qi) and circulates two to three feet outside of the body. This is why someone who is "open" can see auras showing the different colors associated with the five organs, as well as stagnations, excesses, and deficiencies present in the body. When the middle Tan Tien and Heart center are closed, it can contribute to the following Heart conditions: edema, the inability to give or receive love, immune system weakness, speech impediments, mental confusion, delirium, mental illness, insomnia, and ulcers in the mouth, to name a few. When open, one has the ability to express their feelings openly and with clear communication. One will be empathetic, mentally settled, and able to love and be loved. There will also be a heightened awareness around the universal love that exists between all beings.

LOCATION OF THE MIDDLE TAN TIEN

The middle Tan Tien is composed of four points, making the shape of a diamond when all four are connected in the Heart center. One points to the Earth, another to Heaven, and the remaining two connect the front and back of the body.

The first point of the middle Tan Tien is located at CV 12, right below the sternum on the xiphoid process, in the midline of the abdomen. This is the master point for the Middle Burner. This area is sometimes called the Yellow Court Region and reflects emotions stored in the Heart, especially anger, resentment, worry, pensiveness, anxiety, and grief.

The upper front point of the middle Tan Tien is located at CV 22 on the throat. The upper back point is located at GV 14, the Big Bone point, and the lower back point at GV 6, on the middle spine. This is sometimes referred to as the "back gate" to the third chakra.

The center of the middle Tan Tien is in the right atrium of the heart, between the SA (sinoatrial) and the AV (atrioventricular) nodes. The front center point is located at CV 17, in the middle of the sternum at the level of the fourth intercostal space. Also known as the Place of Worship, it is where the Shen (Spirit) is located. This is a major connecting point for the Heart, Lungs, and Pericardium. The back center point (GV 11) is located two inches from the shoulder blades at the fifth or sixth thoracic vertebrae.

The color red is associated with the middle Tan Tien. The healing sound for this region is that of the Heart, "HAAA."

The Upper Tan Tien (Upper Field of Elixir)

The upper Tan Tien is the collector of Heavenly Qi and represents the spiritual aspect of existence and humankind's connection to the divine. This area is considered the Sea of Light; the color associated with it is white. The upper Tan Tien is more of an ethereal-like vapor, connecting with the third level of Wei Qi and our psychic intuition.

When the upper Tan Tien is open, a person will develop an all-knowingness; meaning, they will have foresight and a "knowing" of things that are and yet to come. Some people may equate this to hearing a voice or communicating with God. This area is in connection with the brain and controls memory, hormones, concentration, sight, hearing, touch, and smell—which are in close communication with the Heart and Shen. The brain is referred to as the Sea of Marrow (Sui) and is one of the six Extraordinary Organs. Deficiencies or blockages of the Sea of Marrow may lead to poor memory, cognitive disability, tinnitus, Meniere's disease, Alzheimer's, dementia, and migraines, as well as a lack of spiritual connection, feeling blocked spiritually, and a tendency to blame God for the troubles in our lives, to name a few.

LOCATION OF THE UPPER TAN TIEN

There are three main points that comprise the upper Tan Tien. When all points are connected, it makes the shape of a pyramid collecting the light of the universe. The front point is Yintang, the Hall of Impression point, and represents wisdom and enlightenment. It is also referred to as the third eye.

The back point is located below the external occipital protuberance at GV 16 (Feng Fu), also connected with and surrounded by UB 10 (Heavenly Pillar point). These points act like antennae for receiving messages, and GV 16 is a Sea of Marrow point allowing for the smooth flow of Qi and Blood to the brain; it is a Window of Heaven point used for Shen, or Mind, disturbances.

The top point at GV 20 (Bai Hui), the Hundred Meetings point, was named so because of its connection to receiving divine messages and spiritual intuition. The center of the upper Tan Tien is in the pineal gland, where the Shen emerges with the Wuji, or nothingness. The sound to open up this chamber is "OMM."

The Practice

1. Begin standing in Wuji posture.

2. Allow yourself to become calm and centered.

3. Establish a connection to the Divine, allowing the Bai Hui at the crown of your head to open completely, letting universal energy penetrate the upper Tan Tien.

4. Raise your arms and inhale (like you're Pulling Down the Heavens but with the palms of the hands facing toward your third eye).

5. Exhale as you slowly lower the hands in front of your body, with palms facing inward.

6. When the hands reach the front of the upper Tan Tien, continue exhaling while you make the sound "OMM," pointing the palms (Lao Gong points) toward your third eye. Imagine the chambers

of the upper Tan Tien opening. You can also imagine the color white filling up into this area.

7. As the hands descend to the chest, make the "HAAA" sound, with the palms facing toward your middle Tan Tien. Imagine the chambers in the region opening up and visualize the color red filling up into your Heart center.

8. When the hands reach the lower Tan Tien, imagine those chambers opening up as well, and visualize the color blue connecting with the physical aspect of your being while making the sound "HAREEM."

9. As you guide the hands down the front of the body, imagine the energy beginning to pour down into your upper Tan Tien, flowing down into your middle Tan Tien, and finally into your lower Tan Tien. Allow the vibration to build and maintain a sense of openness.

10. Repeat the practice 9 to 36 times (in multiples of 9).

CHAPTER 20

GOLDEN PEARL EXERCISE

This practice works with the eight Extraordinary Meridians and helps collect nurturing Yin energy from the Earth. As we discussed before, a lot of the eight Extraordinary Vessels are not independent acupuncture meridians; for example, there are Yin and Yang linking vessels, a Yin Stepping Vessel and a Yang Stepping Vessel. These channels are composed of other acupuncture meridians. With this moving Qigong practice, we are stimulating those Eight Extraordinary Vessels. In the next chapter, I will teach you two versions of the Macrocosmic Orbit Meditation. The first is intended to be incorporated with this Golden Pearl practice and is a little more involved with which way energy flows. The second is simplified and can be done separately from this practice. Once you're comfortable with these movements, you can incorporate the first version of the Macrocosmic Orbit Meditation.

This is a simple practice that will leave your body feeling a buzz of energy. While going through the steps, I want you to imagine you are grabbing Yin energy from the Earth. The ancients in Chinese philosophy and medicine believed Earth energy relates back to the Spleen, Stomach, and pancreas. Therefore, as we gather the golden pearl from Earth, we are going to imagine it is yellow. Besides working with the Eight Extraordinary Vessels, this practice is great for grounding and centering oneself. Repeat it between 9 and 36 times (in multiples of 9), or whatever feels good for you.

The Practice

1. Start in Wuji posture with the breath, long, steady, and even, directed deep into the lower Tan Tien.

2. Pull Down the Heavens three times.

3. Inhale and imagine you are scooping up Earth energy with the palms of your hands like you're lifting a giant golden pearl.

4. Once the hands reach about chest height, exhale and expand your arms as if wrapping them around a tree. Imagine the golden pearl expanding between your arms, with both palms facing each other.

5. Inhale and imagine you are squeezing the golden pearl and letting it press into your chest. Then, with both palms facing forward, imagine you are pushing this golden pearl away.

6. Exhale as you press the ball down with palms facing toward the earth, guiding this energy down through your chest and abdomen.

7. Inhale as your palms and the golden pearl come down to the groin and thigh region.

8. Exhale and allow the energy to flow through your shins and feet to disperse back into the earth.

9. Repeat the practice again, inhaling and imagining you're scooping up Earth energy with the palms facing up toward Heaven like lifting a giant golden pearl, then guiding the energy out and down through your body, back into the earth.

10. Finish by Pulling Down the Heavens three times.

11. Store the energy as a white pearl back in your lower Tan Tien.

· CHAPTER 21 ·

MACROCOSMIC
ORBIT MEDITATION

This version of the Macrocosmic Orbit Meditation can be done in conjunction with the Golden Pearl practice in the previous chapter. It can also be done separately, as a standalone meditation.

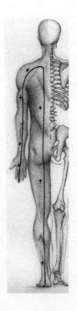
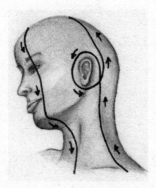

1. Begin this meditation from a standing Wuji posture with the breath long, steady, even and deep, in and out through the nose.

2. Imagine you have pipes that connect to the heels of your feet and travel down to the center of Earth's core.

3. From the heels, imagine the pipes continuing to travel up the back of the legs, then up the back to your Big Bone point (GV 11) at the base of the neck. As you inhale, imagine energy from the Earth rising through the heels and up the pipes to the base of the neck.

4. As you exhale, direct the energy down the outer aspects of the arms, all the way to the tips of your fingers, especially the middle fingers.

5. Take a long inhale, and visualize the energy racing up the inner aspect of your arms, up the neck, circulating around the ears, then to the top of the head.

6. Exhale and imagine this energy flowing down through the front of the face and the chest.

7. Inhale as the energy flows further down your body, through your groin and the top of the thighs.

8. Exhale as the energy flows down through your shins and out through the Bubbling Well points at KI 1, going deep into the ground.

9. Repeat the sequence.

10. Do this practice 9 to 36 times (in multiples of 9).

11. Finish by Pulling Down the Heavens three times.

Macrocosmic Orbit Meditation Version 2

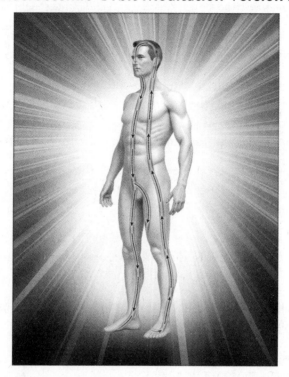

1. From Wuji posture, Pull Down the Heavens three times.

2. Relax and melt down the front, back, and center of your body.

3. Begin breathing into the lower Tan Tien. Imagine it filling up like a balloon with white liquid energy.

4. Allow this energy from the lower Tan Tien to overflow into the perineum (CV 1).

5. Once this occurs, guide the energy down the inside of the legs to the ball of the foot at the Bubbling Well (KI 1) point.

6. Follow the energy up the outside of the legs, bringing Qi back up to the tailbone.

7. Inhale and pull the energy all the way up the spine, along the Governing Vessel, to the top of the head.

8. Exhale and allow the energy to descend down the front of the body along the Conception Vessel and back to the perineum.

9. Next, guide the energy down the inner aspects of the legs, wrapping around the balls of the feet.

10. As you inhale, draw the energy from the outside of the feet up the legs, to the tailbone.

11. Repeat along the Governing Vessel of the spine, up over the top of the head and down the face, chest, and abdomen.

12. Do this practice 9 to 36 times (in multiples of 9).

13. Finish by Pulling Down the Heavens three times.

14. Using visualization, make sure to pull all the energy out of the head and place it back into your lower Tan Tien.

CHAPTER 22

PULLING OUT PAST PAIN MEDITATION

Up to this point, I have discussed how negative emotions get stuck in different organs of the body and create various forms of inflammation, chronic pain, and disease. If you've ever heard the saying, "the issues are in our tissues," this meditation can allow you to feel where you store past, present, and future trauma and events deep in the tissues.

In clinical practice, we see both organ and channel pathology. For example, as I mention in my book, *Chris Shelton's Easy Guide to Fix Neck and Back Pain*, the majority of frozen shoulder, neck pain, and cervical issues are due to emotions that affect the Heart and Lungs. The way we remedy this in-clinic is to work on acupuncture points along the neck that are directly or indirectly related to the Heart and Lungs, opening and releasing the channel pathology. This technique also frees up the stuck emotions that caused the neck or cervical pain to show up in the first place. A lot of times in-clinic, when I touch these points, a majority of my clients have an emotional release and start crying. Once this release occurs, the DNA of the body kicks in and healing begins in the area and tissues affected by the emotional circumstance.

The Practice

1. Go through the Center and Balance Meditation to relax and center yourself.

2. From a seated position, think of something that has caused you pain in the past and/or any type of trauma, either emotional, physical, or both. Really do your best to bring to mind what that experience felt like, bringing into awareness who or what was involved, in addition to any sounds or smells that will further connect you to this past trauma or pain.

3. Next, point to the area where you feel this pain and circle the size and shape where the discomfort is being stored.

4. Now focus on something in the present (i.e. the instructor's voice or any sounds that may be in the room) and point to the area where you feel it. Circle the shape and size of where you are storing the present event.

5. Next, think of something in the future, something upcoming (i.e. a project or event you're excited about but that may cause you worry and anxiety). Again, feel it deeply and point to the area in your body where you sense the present event, circling its size and shape.

6. Bring your awareness back into the area you were storing past pain. Using your mind's intent, begin to push the sensation outside of your body; watch it leave like a dark umbilical cord ascending toward the heavens. As it leaves your body, negative energy is replaced with pure, heavenly, healing energy that fills the space past pain was being stored in.

7. Now, with the negative past experience in front of you, separate the positive from the negative energy (positive energy being wisdom or knowledge learned from the experience), and allow that energy to reside within the body while the negative energy continues to float away toward the heavens.

8. Imagine a sword from Heaven coming down and cutting the negative energy from your body, cutting the painful umbilical cord that tied you to this experience.

9. Now that it has been cut off from your body, visualize the negative energy floating upward toward the heavens. Once it reaches Heaven, see it burst into a shower of golden-white light that falls and engulfs your body. Feel the golden-white light penetrate deep within, healing the wound of past pain and filling your Heart with peace and love.

10. To finish this practice, center yourself by Pulling Down the Heavens three times, storing the energy in the lower Tan Tien.

CHAPTER 23

WRAPPING THE WAIST

The Wrapping the Waist practice is great for stimulating the Kidneys and certain acupuncture points on the arms, waist, chest, and rib cage. This practice also stimulates one of the eight Extraordinary Vessels, called the Belt, or Girdle, Vessel. The Belt Vessel is the only horizontal acupuncture meridian in the body. This channel encompasses the three Yin and Yang channels of the legs. A lot of cases I see in-clinic for pain in the lower back, sciatica, hip, and tailbone are due to Belt Channel blockage or tightness. This channel begins at the Ming Men (GV 4) on the spine, encircles the waist like a belt connecting to Liver 13 on the free-floating rib, then dips down into the anterior abdominal region and across the posterior lumbar region. It connects with Gallbladder 26, 27, and 28 points and crosses the Conception Vessel in the front of the body above the pubic bone around CV 3.

Girdle Vessel

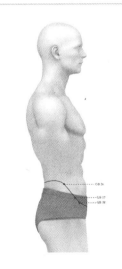

A byproduct of this practice enables the energy of the body to increase through Qi cultivation. Qi within the Belt Vessel strengthens the body's defense mechanism, the Wei Qi. This practice also helps stimulate and strengthen the Kidneys while loosening up the lower lumbar region. It is helpful for anyone with a cold, flu, or cough, as well as anyone who is experiencing grief or sadness.

The Practice

1. Begin this meditation from a standing Wuji posture with the breath long, even, and deep, filling into the lower Tan Tien.

2. With your feet shoulder-with apart, begin to twist the upper torso and allow the arms and hands to swing freely.

3. As the hands wrap around the waist on the back, have the back of the hand tap the kidneys on the left and right sides of the spine.

4. When the arms swing around to the front, have your hands pat either your chest, opposite arm, or rib cage.

5. Use your legs as a pump to shift your weight from left to right, which will further help the upper torso to move freely. This movement stimulates your lymphatic system and increases blood flow to your heart.

6. If you suffer from chronic grief, sadness, cough, cold, or flu, have your hands pat the LU 1 and 2 points on your chest (where the chest muscle meets the shoulder).

7. If you have a Spleen deficiency, as the hands wrap around to the front, have them tap the sides of your rib cage at SP 21 (about 1 to 2 inches below your armpit).

8. If you have Liver Qi stagnation, digestive issues, bloating, abdominal distention, or moodiness, tap LV 13, LV 14, GB 24, and SP 16 on the lower part of your rib cage.

9. Do this practice for 5 to 10 minutes, or whatever amount of time feels comfortable for you.

10. Finish by Pulling Down the Heavens three times and storing the energy in the lower Tan Tien.

CHAPTER 24

FIVE DIRECTION MEDITATION

This meditation connects us with the five directions and the five Yin Yang organs system. It is sometimes called the Wu Zang meditation. The words Wu and Zang relate to the Zang Fu organ system. "Zang," meaning organ, and "Fu," pertaining to five. The theories of Classical Chinese medicine can't emphasize enough the importance of optimal functioning of all five Yin organs. Referring to chapter 6 and the Five Elements, the text covers many of the different aspects each element connects, or relates, to. The ancients understood, through observation and study, the importance of the five directions and how the 28 constellations, the North Star, and the five planets Mercury, Venus, Saturn, Jupiter, and Mars influence our physiology, health, psychology, and overall experience on this planet.

The purpose of this meditation is to add another layer of assistance in cleansing the body, rectifying physical and emotional imbalances while strengthening our bodies against the invasion of external pathogens, like the common cold or flu.

The original energy of the universe is incomprehensible. Some call "It" God, Oneness, or Universal Consciousness. Words can point to but cannot fully describe It. There is no differentiation—everything is absolute, whole, and complete. It is beyond time and space, exhibiting existence and nonexistence simultaneously. This ethereal nothingness was called Wuji by ancient Chinese philosophers. It is said that Wuji is the origin of the creation of Heaven and Earth.

In Chinese cosmology, compass directions were developed to be south facing. So, in this practice, we will begin by facing south. Because the sun rises in the east (Yang) and sets in the west (Yin), when we face south, east will be on our left and west on our right.

Wu Zang Meditation

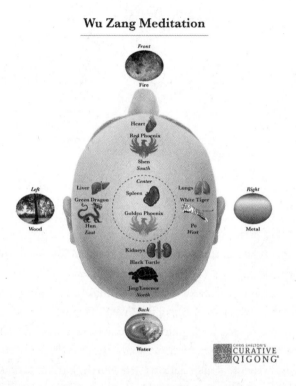

The Practice

1. This meditation can be done from a seated or standing Wuji posture. Begin by Pulling Down the Heavens three times, allowing the breath to flow deep into the lower abdomen, or lower Tan Tien.

2. Start by facing the southern direction. Even if it's daylight, imagine connecting with the starry constellations in the south.

3. Begin by imagining the constellations forming the shape of the Red Phoenix, connecting to your Heart. Visualize a red glow emanating from the Red Phoenix that begins to envelop and descend the entire front of your body. Imagine the front of your body covered with this red light.

4. Now connect with the stars to the right of you, on the western horizon. The starry constellations in the west form the shape of the White Tiger. Imagine a white glow emanating from the White Tiger that begins to envelop and descend the entire right side of your body, connecting to your Lungs. See this area immersed in white light as you connect with the western stars of White Tiger.

5. Move your attention to the stars behind you, connecting with the northern horizon.

6. The starry constellations in the north form the shape of the Blue Turtle. Imagine a blue glow emanating from the Blue Turtle that begins to envelop and descend the entire back side of your body, connecting to your Kidneys. Once you have immersed the entire back of your body with the starry energy from Blue Turtle, everything on your backside radiates its blue color.

7. Now connect with the stars to the left of you, on the eastern horizon. The starry constellations in the east form the shape of the Green Dragon. Imagine an emerald green glow emanating from the Green Dragon that begins to envelop and descend the entire left side of your body while also connecting to your Liver. See this area become emerald green as you connect with the eastern stars of Green Dragon.

8. Connect now with the Golden Phoenix above and below the Earth, relating to the Spleen. Feel everything that is facing down, and imagine a golden light radiating through the center of your body, going deep into the Earth, illuminating and touching everything in its path.

9. Next, imagine the Red Phoenix begins to chase the White Tiger on the right, which in turn chases the Blue Turtle at the back. The Blue Turtle then chases the Green Dragon to the left, completing the cycle as the Green Dragon follows the Red Phoenix in this circular form.

10. Imagine these animals and their associated colors and constellations chasing one another as they move in a clockwise direction. The animals are spinning around you so fast, you can no longer

differentiate one from the next. The colors begin to merge into one another as they spin faster, and faster.

11. Continue until everything is moving so fast that you find yourself standing in a space of emptiness and brilliant white light. Allow this state of being-ness to continue for several heartbeats.

12. Then, watch as the clockwise motion slows, and you begin to see the colors of the four directions become visible. You can now see, once again, the Red Phoenix chasing the White Tiger, the White Tiger chasing the Blue Turtle, the Blue Turtle chasing the Green Dragon, and the Green Dragon chasing the Red Phoenix.

13. Continue to watch as it slows until all motion has come to a stop.

14. Now we move in a counterclockwise direction, starting from the south and the Red Phoenix. This time, the Red Phoenix starts by chasing the Green Dragon. The Green Dragon chases the Blue Turtle, the Blue Turtle chases the White Tiger, and the White Tiger chases Red Phoenix as the cycle continues.

15. Again, watch the energies as they begin to circulate with increasing speed, all directions moving faster and faster as one follows the other.

16. Come into a place where you can no longer differentiate the distinct shades, the Red Phoenix from the Green Dragon, the Blue Turtle from the White Tiger; see the colors start to blend together as one until the movement is so fast, you once again find yourself standing in a space of emptiness and brilliant white light.

17. Feel into this state of being-ness for several heartbeats.

18. Then, as before, the counterclockwise motion begins to slow, and you see the colors of the four directions as they return to view.

19. You notice, once again, the Red Phoenix chasing the Green Dragon, the Green Dragon chasing the Blue Turtle, the Blue Turtle chasing the White Tiger, and the White Tiger completing the cycle by chasing the Red Phoenix. See them as they continue to slow, until all motion has come to a stop.

20. At this point, you should feel energized and expansive.

21. End this meditation by Pulling Down the Heavens three times, storing the energy back into the lower Tan Tien.

Purification for the Body

The following is an invocation by Taoist Master, Hua Ching Ni, from his book, *Workbook for Spiritual Development*. This invocation brings forth a response from the subtle universal realms, the five directions, and the constellations as a means to further strengthen your vitality and protect you from external pathogenic factors or psychic attacks from others.

To properly recite this invocation, position yourself in a comfortable and quiet environment. Inhale at the beginning of each sentence, and exhale as you read it through, repeating with the next. Do this for the entire invocation.

With the sun, I wash my body.
With the moon, I refine my form.
With the divine immortals, I am supported.
With the eternal beings, I perpetuate my own eternal life.
I unite myself with the enduring energy of the twenty-eight constellations.
Within and without, all impurities are cleansed with divine water.
Most respected heavenly divinity, console my body.
Saturate my soul's energy with the light of all stars in the enormous "bushel"
    of space.
Eastern stars of the "Green Dragon,"
lead me forward.
Western stars of the "White Tiger,"
protect me from behind.
Southern stars of the "Red Bird,"
guard me from above.
Northern stars of the "Blue Turtle,"
guard me from below.
So, it is commanded and confirmed.

CHAPTER 25

THREE TAN TIEN CLEANSING EXERCISE

In chapter 19, Opening the Three Tan Tiens, the focus was on connecting with these three major Seas of Energy in order to release any physical, mental, or spiritual blockages. This is done while simultaneously increasing the function of our body by harmonizing all three of these spheres in coordination with the internal organs and their associated acupuncture meridians. This next practice goes deeper into cleansing each of the three Tan Tiens individually.

As seen in the image below, the upper Tan Tien radiates light and the middle emanates electricity, magnetism, and sound. It influences what is referred to as Stomach Fire and Heart Fire. Stomach Fire relates to rotting and ripening during the transformation and transportation of food essence and fluid sent up to the chest to be made into Blood. Heart Fire relates to our Mind and Spirit. When functioning properly, a person's mind will be settled, the eyes glistening, and the spirit intact. The lower Tan Tien emanates generated heat, and is also responsible for Bladder and Kidney Fire. Bladder Fire plays an essential role in transforming bodily fluids into Qi, as well as in the separation of pure fluids from the impure, sending pure fluids up to the chest and those that are impure out of the body in the form of urine. Kidney Fire is equally important, creating a "steam" in the form of Qi that circulates throughout the body. You may notice that while doing this practice, you develop a lot of internal heat. This is normal and a result of diving deeper into your cleansing journey.

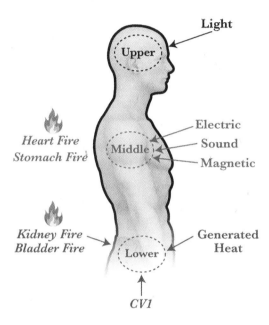

Three Tan Tiens

The Practice

1. This practice can be done from a seated or standing Wuji posture. Begin by Pulling Down the Heavens three times, allowing the breath to be long, steady, even, and deep into the lower Tan Tien.

2. Gently begin to shift your weight from left to right.

3. As you shift your weight to the right, inhale while bringing the left palm up to the third eye in between the eyebrows.

4. Exhale as you shift back to the left, pulling the palm away like you're flinging away dark energy from the third eye.

5. Inhale; the right palm moves in front of the third eye. As you shift toward the right, exhale and imagine the right palm is further

pulling out dark, stagnant energy from the upper Tan Tien (the third eye).

6. As the right palm is flinging turbid energy to the right, the left palm is now facing toward the third eye. Repeat the steps listed above, switching side to side.

7. Each time you pull the hands away, imagine you are peeling away any dark layers that might be obstructing your connection with your higher self, or God.

8. As you continue to remove the blockages and toxins from the upper Tan Tien, see a brilliant white pearl emerge. Watch as it shines behind your third eye, or upper Tan Tien.

9. Repeat this action 9 to 36 times (in multiples of 9).

10. Next, place your palms in front of your middle Tan Tien, in the center of your chest at the level of your Heart.

11. Inhale as you shift the weight to the right, bringing the left palm up to your Heart center.

12. Exhale and shift back to the left, pulling the palm away like you're flinging dark energy, abandonment, and emotional pain away from your Heart center.

13. Inhale; the right palm moves in front of your Heart center.

14. Exhale as you shift toward the right, pulling the right palm away while imagining it is further pulling out dark, stagnant energy or emotional pain from your Heart center.

15. As the right palm flings turbid energy to the right, the left palm is now facing toward the Heart center. Continue the practice side to side.

16. Now, as you pull the hands away, imagine you are peeling away any dark layers that are keeping your Heart from being open.

17. As you continue to remove the blockages and toxins from the middle Tan Tien, watch as a crimson red pearl shines brightly in the center of your chest.

18. Repeat this action 9 to 36 times (in multiples of 9).

19. Now place your palms in front of your lower Tan Tien, in the lower abdominal region, below the navel.

20. Inhale as you shift the weight to the right, bringing the left palm up to your lower Tan Tien.

21. Exhale and shift back to the left, pulling the palm away like you're flinging away dark energy, physical limitations, or pain from the lower Tan Tien.

22. Inhale as the right palm moves in front of your lower Tan Tien. Exhale as you shift toward the right, imagining the right palm is further pulling out dark, stagnant energy or physical trauma from the lower Tan Tien.

23. As the right palm is flinging the turbid energy to the right, the left palm now is facing toward the lower Tan Tien. Continue the practice from side to side.

24. This time, as you pull the hands away, imagine you are peeling away any dark layers obstructing you from being able to enjoy physical activities you once did or other limitations keeping you from breaking through a challenge or obstacle in your life.

25. As you continue to remove blockages and toxins from the lower Tan Tien, watch as a cobalt blue pearl now shines brightly from the lower abdominal region.

26. Repeat this action 9 to 36 times (in multiples of 9).

27. Pause and feel any sensations now arising from these three energy centers.

28. Finish by Pulling Down the Heavens three times, collecting the energy and storing it back into the lower Tan Tien.

CHAPTER 26

SUN AND MOON MEDITATION

The Sun and Moon Meditation helps balance the Yin and Yang aspects of our being. It is also used to harmonize Yin Yang diseases and pathology. This meditation detoxifies emotional stagnation and establishes physical, emotional, and spiritual well-being. The sun is considered Yang, and the moon, Yin.

In chapter 39, I've inserted a Yin and Yang Typology Questionnaire. One of the ways this practice can be beneficial is when you're too much of either polarity. If a dominant Yang type, the lunar meditation will increase Yin energy, balancing out excessive Yang, and vice versa. If excessively Yin, the solar meditation will balance this by increasing Yang energy. In Classical Chinese medicine, there are many different types of diseases that have their roots in Yin Yang imbalance. Please refer to my book, *Chris Shelton's Easy Guide to Fix Neck and Back Pain* for more information. In this book, I detail the symptoms of dis-ease that manifest when Yin and Yang are out of balance.

The two most common conditions seen in-clinic are Yin and Yang deficiency. Some of the symptoms of Yin deficiency include night sweats, eye or facial tremors, pain that migrates throughout the body, and a feeling that your body is hot without a rise in temperature. Besides diet, herbal recommendations, and other Qigong practices, the lunar meditation can be quite helpful in offsetting these symptoms. Some signs of Yang deficiency include feeling cold or having cold extremities, watery stool, undigested food in the stool, edema, and frequent, pale urination. Practicing the solar meditation along with dietary changes can be helpful in reducing these symptoms.

The best time to practice the moon, or lunar, meditation is three days before the full moon, the day of the full moon, and/or three days after the full moon. This is when you will receive the most abundant supply of lunar Yin energy. Though it is also beneficial to practice this meditation using your imagination, looking directly at the moon is best. If it's too cold outside, I suggest practicing indoors while looking at the moon through a window. This will help limit the possibility of an invasion of Wind Cold, manifesting as symptoms of the common cold or flu.

The best time to practice the sun, or solar, meditation is right before sunrise during the summer months and after sunrise during winter months. Please be careful not to look at the sun directly; instead, have a soft, unfocused gaze. Even though I am a Yang dominant type, I find the solar meditation is very helpful when my Qi feels weak or deficient. I will also utilize this practice when I feel that my energy is a little bit off from not getting enough sleep the night before.

The Practice

Sun/Solar Meditation:

1. This practice can be done from a seated or standing Wuji posture.

2. Begin this practice by Pulling Down the Heavens three times, allowing the breath to be long, steady, even, and deep into the lower Tan Tien.

3. Facing the sun, have a soft, unfocused gaze.

4. Reaching toward the sun, imagine you can grab it and pull its warming Yang energy into the eyes and the Crown Point at the top of the head (GV 20).

5. Imagine the rays of the warm sun filling into the upper Tan Tien. As you exhale, with palms facing the third eye, swallow. Using your hands, guide the solar energy down through the middle and into the lower Tan Tien.

6. Repeat several times, each time imagining the sun getting brighter and brighter, filling up all three of your energy centers.

7. Finish this practice by placing the hands on the lower abdomen and feel the sun's warmth radiate from the lower Tan Tien, filling up into all the tissues of the body.

8. Relax and Pull Down the Heavens three times, making sure to pull any excess Qi out of the head.

Moon/Lunar Meditation:

1. This practice can be done from a seated or standing Wuji posture.

2. Begin this practice by Pulling Down the Heavens three times, allowing the breath to be long, steady, even, and deep into the lower Tan Tien.

3. Gaze toward the moon and allow its nurturing Yin energy to penetrate the eyes, the third eye, and the Crown Point on the top of the head (GV 20).

4. Reach toward the moon, and imagine you can grab it and pull its cooling Yin energy into the eyes and the Crown Point.

5. Imagine the moon's light filling into your upper Tan Tien.

6. As you exhale, with palms facing the third eye, swallow. Using your hands, guide the lunar energy down through the middle and into the lower Tan Tien.

7. Now imagine the full moon's light radiating within all three energy centers.

8. Repeat this several times, imagining the moon getting brighter and brighter as it fills these energy centers.

9. Finish the practice by placing the hands on the lower abdomen and feel the moon's cooling, nurturing energy radiate from the lower Tien into all of tissues of the body.

10. Relax and Pull Down the Heavens three times, sure pull any excess Qi out of the head.

· CHAPTER 27 ·

BONE-CLEANSING
MEDITATION

This book covers various practices to help rid the body of toxins and emotional buildup. We started from the superficial layers by Brushing the Meridians to stimulate the flow of Qi. We then moved through the Yin Organ Cleansing exercises to cleanse the body's internal organs, namely the Heart, Spleen, Lungs, Kidneys, and Liver. This was followed by purifying the vital energy centers of the body, the three Seas of Energy, the Tan Tiens. The next, more profound, layer of healing involves cleansing deep into the marrow and bone. According to CCM, the bones and marrow are considered Extraordinary Organs due to their role in storing precious Yin Essence.

As in western medicine, the bones are responsible for the production of blood. They are considered the cavity that houses marrow and are connected directly to the Kidneys. The marrow of the bone nourishes the brain and spinal cord, and because Post-Heaven Qi plays a crucial role in its production, proper diet, nutrition, and what we put into our bodies will affect the strength and quality of the marrow.

According to Chinese medicine, Kidney Essence nourishes bone marrow and provides structure to the bones. Therefore, if Kidney Essence is weak, the marrow and bones will lose this nourishment, and the bones may become brittle. In extreme cases, a person may lose the ability to stand or walk. To speed up the healing of bone fractures, you can tonify and strengthen the Kidneys and the Kidney channel. This can be accomplished with the Wrapping the Waist and Kidney Cleansing exercises. The Kidney Healing Sound meditation will further help to support this healing process.

Many different layers comprise the bones, which have two distinct regions: the diaphysis and the epiphysis. The diaphysis is the hollow tubular shaft that runs from one end of the bone to the other. The outer layer of the diaphysis is called the cortical bone, and the endosteum is composed of the lining of the bone adjacent to the medullary cavity (where marrow is located). As you become more familiar with the following meditation, imagine feeling into these different layers of the bone and marrow, each time going deeper and deeper.

After the first couple of times doing this practice, it is normal for the body to ache the following day, almost like you have the flu. This is due to the powerful cleansing effect it has on the bones and marrow.

This practice can help to enhance the endocrine system and Central Nervous System (CNS) as well as relieve certain blood disorders. It may be

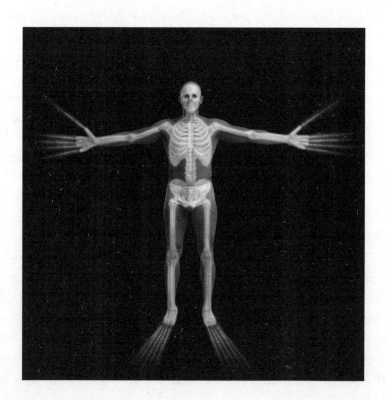

helpful for the early onset of bone degeneration, Alzheimer's, dementia, certain types of cancers, and osteoporosis. As with all Qigong practices in this book, check with your primary care physician if you have been diagnosed with any of these conditions before implementing this practice into your routine.

The following is based on an exercise found in *The Essence of Internal Martial Arts*, Volumes 1 and 2, by Jerry Alan Johnson.

The Practice

Step 1

1. Begin this meditation from a seated or standing Wuji posture, allowing the breath to penetrate long, steady, even, and deep into the lower Tan Tien.

2. Pull Down the Heavens three times to settle your mind.

3. Relax the hands and feet, allowing the fingers and toes to widen. This will open the PC 8 point on the palms and the KI 1 point on the bottoms of the feet.

4. Inhale and visualize the color black (as in water or a mist) penetrating into the hands and feet through the fingers, toes, PC 8, and KI 1 points. Watch as it travels up through the bones of the body, finally pulling the energy up above the skull.

5. As you prepare to exhale, starting at the top of the head, imagine you are now pushing the black water or mist down through the crown of the head into the skeletal system, washing the bones and marrow as it passes through the body.

6. Upon exhalation, direct this dark fluid or mist down through the bones and out the fingertips, toes, PC 8, and KI 1 points. Visualize the toxic buildup being washed out of the bones and marrow as it passes through them. In this process, see how the water or mist has changed in color; it now appears dull, or cloudy, as it cleans the bones and marrow of built-up toxins and impurities.

7. As you visualize this washing process, be sure to feel deeply into the experience. Notice the sensations of cleansing deep into the bones and marrow of the entire body.

8. Next, watch as the bones turn gray in the areas where the black mist or fluid has passed through. Do this until the entire skeletal structure becomes a solid gray color throughout.

Step 2

1. Now going deeper into the bone marrow, once again inhale through the bones, all the way to the top of the head.

2. As you prepare to exhale, imagine you will now be pushing the color gray down and out through the skeletal system.

3. While exhaling, imagine the gray color passing through the bones and marrow, carrying any remaining toxins out as it leaves the fingertips, toes, PC 8, and KI 1 points.

4. Again, you may notice it has changed in color as it further cleanses these deep tissues of the body.

5. Once this is complete, see the skeletal system as it turns a glistening pearl-white in the areas where the gray color has passed through. Do this until the bones of the body radiate a brilliant pearl-white from head to toe.

Step 3

1. Repeat the practice, once again starting with the color black, then gray, ending in pearl-white.

2. Do this exercise 9 to 36 times (in multiples of 9).

3. End the practice by Pulling Down the Heavens three times and storing the energy back into the lower Tan Tien.

CHAPTER 28

FIVE CLOUD MEDITATION

This is probably one of my favorite Qigong cleansing exercises. It combines the five major planets with their associated organs, colors, and healing sounds. I personally feel more when I do this practice inaudibly, making the healing sounds underneath my breath. For the purposes of this practice, we are going to start off by doing the sounds audibly as we connect with the five planets.

PLANET	ORGAN		COLOR	HEALING SOUND
Jupiter	Liver	Gallbladder	Green	SHUUU
Mars	Heart	Small Intestines	Red	HAAAA
Saturn	Spleen	Stomach	Yellow	HUUUU
Venus	Lungs	Large Intestines	White	SSSSS
Mercury	Kidneys	Urinary Bladder	Blue	FUUUU

- ☯ The planet Jupiter connects with the Liver and Gallbladder; the color is green.

- ☯ The planet Mars connects with the Heart and Small Intestine; the color is red.

- ☯ The planet Saturn connects with the Spleen and Stomach; the color is yellow.

- ☯ The planet Venus connects with the Lungs and Large Intestine; the color is white.

- ☯ The planet Mercury connects with the Kidneys and Urinary Bladder; the color is blue.

The Practice

1. Begin this meditation from a seated or standing Wuji posture, allowing the breath to penetrate long, steady, even, and deep into the lower Tan Tien.

2. Pull Down the Heavens three times to settle your mind.

3. Imagine connecting with the planets Jupiter, Mars, Saturn, Venus, and Mercury.

4. See a green cloud surrounding Jupiter, a red cloud surrounding Mars, a yellow cloud surrounding Saturn, a white cloud surrounding Venus, and a blue cloud surrounding Mercury.

5. Visualize all these clouds coming together and entering into the Bai Hui (GV 20) at the Crown Point on the top of the head.

6. The clouds glide down to the Liver and Gallbladder on the right side of your body and envelop these two organs while they come together, turning a brilliant emerald green color.

7. Bring to mind a circumstance, past or present, that creates anger, resentment, or irritation for you. Feel into your body as if it is happening now. Who's involved? What's involved?

8. As you inhale, pull the emerald green cloud into the area of your Liver. Exhale, making the "SHUU" (shh-ooo) sound and allow that

circumstance to leave like a dark cloud, going several feet away from your body and deep into the ground.

9. Continue to make the "SHUU" sound for several breaths, releasing the anger and frustration with each exhale, allowing the positive virtues of kindness and creativity to come in their place.

10. Next, allow the emerald green cloud to ascend to the Heart. Once it reaches the Heart center, see it change into a beautiful crimson red color.

11. Focusing on the emotions of abandonment, loneliness, or lack of joy, allow this cloud to penetrate deep into the muscle of the heart.

12. As you exhale, make the healing sound of "HAAA," and watch as the sorrowful emotions leave like a dark cloud going several feet away from your body and deep into the ground.

13. Do this for several breaths, letting go of the trauma and pain, bringing forth the positive virtue of love to fill the space.

14. Next, guide the red cloud as it descends to the Spleen on the left side of your body.

15. Once this red cloud reaches the Spleen, watch as it turns a bright canary yellow, penetrating deep into the organ and surrounding region.

16. Focusing on the negative emotions of worry, over-intellectualizing and anxiety, bring to mind a situation, event, or person that triggers these emotions.

17. As you inhale, pull the canary yellow cloud deep into the Spleen. Exhale, making the "HUUU" (hhh-ooo) sound, allowing that circumstance to leave like a dark cloud going several feet away from your body and deep into the ground.

18. Do this for several breaths. As we let go of worry and anxiety, the positive virtues of peace of mind and serenity take their place.

19. Now allow this canary yellow cloud to ascend up the chest and envelop the Lungs, where it becomes a bright pearl-white.

20. Focusing on the emotions of grief, sadness, disappointment, shame, and guilt, visualize this pearl-white cloud sinking deeper and deeper into the Lungs.

21. Exhale, making the healing sound of "SSSS," allowing these emotions to leave like a dark cloud going several feet away from the body and deep into the ground.

22. Do this for several breaths. As we let go of grief and sorrow, this pearl-white cloud penetrates deep into the Lungs, bringing forth the positive virtue of courage.

23. Next, allow this pearl-white cloud to descend to the Kidneys on the low back, opposite the navel.

24. Once this pearl-white cloud reaches the Kidneys, watch as it turns a brilliant cobalt blue.

25. Focusing on the negative emotions of fear or shock, bring up any situation, past or present, that triggers these for you.

26. As you inhale, pull the blue cloud deep into the Kidneys. Exhale making the "FUUU" sound, allowing this circumstance to leave like a dark cloud going several feet away from your body and deep into the ground.

27. Do this for several breaths. As we let go of fear and shock, the positive virtues of gentleness, wisdom, and willpower come forth.

28. Finally, allow yourself to visualize the different colored clouds surrounding the five main organs. Then, imagine the cloud of each color associated with its corresponding planet.

29. Watch as these clouds ascend up and out through the Crown Point, returning to their planets.

30. Take a moment to thank the planets for their wisdom and gifts of healing.

31. Finish the practice by Pulling Down the Heavens three times and storing the energy back in the lower Tan Tien.

CHAPTER 29

STAYING PRESENT

By now, I hope you have taken the first steps in establishing your Qigong practice. The White Pearl Meditation is particularly helpful for replenishing your life battery, the Kidneys. The Center and Balance Meditation is an excellent technique for keeping yourself centered and grounded. You have also learned to Brush the Meridians to keep energy flowing through them. The Microcosmic and Macrocosmic Orbit Meditations will lead you deeper and deeper into awareness of the ebb and flow of Qi within your body. In addition, you have learned the five exercises to harmonize key Yin organs, one for each of the Five Elements. The Five Cloud and Five Direction Meditations, as well as the Six Healing Sounds will assist you in diving deeper into releasing past trauma. Most importantly of all, I hope you have learned to be present in your body. The mental world constantly lures us with hopes, fears, regrets, and thoughts of past and future, but our life is here, in the now. Your body, your very own Qi, can be one of the most exciting parts of your own universe.

I hope, too, that in doing these exercises, you have experienced some benefit. Maybe not much, and maybe not every time, but enough to show you the value of them, and make you want to continue. As with any other human activity, getting the full benefit demands that you DO IT, ideally, on a regular basis.

In the next section, I will describe three different daily routines—a full routine for those with time and dedication (1 to 2 hours), a 20-minute routine, and a 1-minute routine. For everyone, I recommend doing the Renewal of Spirit Meditation (described below) each week on Sunday. As with every other part of the cosmos, our energies function rhythmically and cyclically. Yang energy begins to build from Sunday, peaks on Wednesday, then declines as Yin energy builds. Thus, Sunday is that "still point" where we can pause, reestablish our center, and express our intention for the week. (It may also be a good day for working people to do the full routine if more time is available.) Create a routine that you can realistically meet; persevere with patience, and be confident that results are coming.

Renewal of Spirit Meditation

This meditation can be done daily or once a week, ideally on Sunday, to renew your Qi for the coming week. It is also ideal during any seasonal change, such as the spring or vernal equinoxes. You can begin with invocations, prayer, and/or an energy cultivation practice, or you may simply begin.

1. As usual, start with the Three Regulations: steady breath, relaxed mind, Wuji posture (feet shoulder-width apart, shoulders relaxed and broad, tailbone tucked, Crown Point rising).

2. Pull Down the Heavens three times.

3. Allow heavenly energy to descend. As this divine Qi descends, imagine that any and all dark, turbid Qi from the body is pushed out through the feet and sent deep into the earth.

4. Start the Mystical Pearl Meditation: Focusing on your breathing, breathe deeply into the lower Tan Tien for five minutes. Imagine it filling with golden, mystical light from the Earth.

5. Now bring your awareness to the Third Eye in the center of the forehead, the upper Tan Tien, and imagine a brown pearl turning there. Feel this brown pearl pulsating, rotating, and vibrating.

6. Next, imagine peeling away the brown skin of this pearl and polishing it until it becomes a brilliant white, shining and filling the entire upper Tan Tien with pure radiance, illuminating all your senses.

7. Next, imagine the white light descending through your body, cleansing everything in its path.

8. Focus on the golden light of the lower Tan Tien and allow the golden and white lights to mix. Feel the mixed energy cleansing every part of your body and emotions.

9. Imagine the cleansing energy moving down. Focus on the bottoms of the feet and visualize turbid energy leaving through the balls of the feet, replaced by pure energy.

10. As you feel your body becoming purified, cleansed, and rejuvenated, start to bring your awareness back to the present.

11. Slowly awaken your sensory organs, one at a time, starting with your ears, allowing them to completely open. Next, stimulate your saliva and the mouth, allowing it to fully awaken. Then, the nose as nasal sensations bring in positive life force energy. Finally, the pores of the skin. Allow the pores to open, bringing in a heightened awareness of everything around you. Feel into your environment and notice a sense of connectedness to everything.

13. Now, simply relax. You are ready to start your day (or week) with increased awareness, alertness, and profound tranquility, grounded and centered in your true nature.

14. To close the practice, Pull Down the Heavens three times.

CHAPTER 30

SUGGESTED DAILY ROUTINES

The Full Routine (1 to 2 hours)

1. Remembering the Three Regulations, assume Wuji posture.

2. Pull Down the Heavens three times.

3. Perform the three Qi Clearing Exercises; finish by Pulling Down the Heavens.

4. Practice the Center and Balance Meditation. (Do this until you can feel the sensation throughout your entire body at once. In the beginning this may take 10 to 14 minutes; later you will achieve it in 1 or 2 minutes.) Pull Down the Heavens three times.

5. Include the Microcosmic and Macrocosmic Orbit Meditations for 5 to 10 minutes each. Pull Down the Heavens three times.

6. Brush the Meridians three times. Pull Down the Heavens three times.

7. Massage the Yang Organs. Pull Down the Heavens three times.

8. Next, the five Yin Organ Cleansing Exercises (Heart, Spleen, Lungs, Kidneys, and Liver). Perform each of the Yin organ exercises beginning with the Heart, the Emperor or Empress of the body. Do each one at least three times; you may add more for any organ you want to target specifically. Pull Down the Heavens three times.

9. Include the Six Healing Sounds and combine these with the Five Direction and Five Cloud Meditations. Pull Down the Heavens three times.

10. Next, the Bone-Cleansing Exercise. Pull Down the Heavens three times.

11. Finish with the White Pearl Meditation, storing the Essence you have gathered in your battery pack, the Kidneys.

20-Minute Routine

1. Remembering the Three Regulations, assume Wuji posture.

2. Pull Down the Heavens three times.

3. Perform the three Qi Clearing Exercises. Finish by Pulling Down the Heavens.

4. Practice the Microcosmic or Macrocosmic Orbit Meditation for 5 to 10 minutes. Pull Down the Heavens three times.

5. Next, the five Yin Organ Cleansing Exercises (Heart, Spleen, Lungs, Kidneys, and Liver). Perform each of the Yin organ exercises beginning with the Heart, the Emperor/Empress of the body. Do each one at least three times; you may add more for any organ you want to target specifically. You may also combine the Six Healing Sounds with the five Yin Organ Exercises. Pull Down the Heavens three times.

6. Finish with the White Pearl Meditation, storing the Essence you have gathered in your battery pack, the Kidneys.

1-Minute Routine

1. Remembering the Three Regulations, assume Wuji posture.

2. Pull Down the Heavens three times.

3. Practice the White Pearl Meditation.

4. Pull Down the Heavens three times.

CHAPTER 31

THE FIVE ELEMENTS QUESTIONNAIRE EXPLAINED

Like other aspects of the world, our own personalities can also be understood in terms of the Five Elements. The Elements are expressed in our dominant emotions, appearance, and personality. They can also be used to predict what diseases we are likely to suffer from. Knowing the strengths and weaknesses of the Elements in your own nature can help you better understand yourself and make life-affirming choices in every sphere of life, from diet to home décor. More broadly, recognizing Element archetypes in others can help you understand them on a deeper, more compassionate level.

In chapter 37, you will find a Five Elements Questionnaire. Take this Questionnaire now to assess your personality in terms of the Five Elements. Are you a Wood Type? A Fire Type? Or a mixture of two? Are you a Fire Type with Metal issues? In future lessons, we will discuss each of the five archetypes in depth. First, simply take the Questionnaire.

Instructions for Taking the Questionnaire

The questions are grouped in five sections, or "phases." Answer according to how you are now—not how you want to be, or how you used to be. If the condition in the question sounds a lot like you, select a +2. If the condition (or attitude) sounds somewhat like you, choose a +1. Conversely, if the question doesn't describe you at all, select −2, or if somewhat, a −1 and a 0 for neutral. Do not get caught up in the details, especially whether it's −1 or −2. When answering the questions, try to avoid overthinking what your answer "should" be. There is no hierarchy in nature's Five Elements. Later, in evaluating your scores, you will be interested in their spread—that is, the highest and lowest scores—not in what is in between.

When you have answered all the questions, add up the count for each phase and arrange them in order from highest to lowest score. Then turn to the Five Elements Questionnaire Answers in Chapter 37 to learn which phase corresponds to each Element; or simply take the questionnaire by scanning the QR code below or visiting www.qigongforemotionalwellbeing.com.

Advice for Interpreting Your Results

This questionnaire will reveal the predominant (highest score) and weakest (lowest score) archetypes, or elements, in your personality. At the beginning, for the sake of keeping things simple, concern yourself only with your predominant and weakest elements. It is possible that your predominant type is a combination—a Metal/Earth type for example—but don't consider that possibility at first.

Your highest score/strongest archetype describes the fundamental way you approach the world. Deviations from your predominant archetype may explain why certain personality traits, habits, and/or health issues affect you. Your lowest score suggests areas of weakness where you might want to focus energy to achieve greater balance and harmony. The descriptions of individual archetypes in later chapters will guide you further in understanding how to do this.

Many factors—including geographic location, diet, lifestyle, habits, etc.—can create variations in these archetypes. These factors can also influence whether the archetype is expressed in a positive or negative way. Remember, too, that your fundamental archetype may change in different stages in your life.

The Five Elements Chart

Element	Fire	Earth	Metal	Water	Wood
Color	Red	Orange Yellow	White	Black Blue	Green
Seasons	Summer	Indian Summer	Autumn	Winter	Spring
Yin organs (Solid Organs)	Heart Pericardium	Spleen	Lungs	Kidneys	Liver
Yang Organs (Hollow Organs)	Small Intestine Triple Burner	Stomach	Large Intestine	Bladder	Gallbladder
Negative Emotions	Over-excitation Mania	Anxiety Worry Overthinking	Sadness Grief Disappointment	Fear Shock PTSD	Anger Resentment Rage
Positive Virtues	Love Gratitude	Balance Centeredness	Courage Inspiration	Gentleness Wisdom	Kindness Creativity
Healing Sounds	Hhhaaa Szzzzz	Hhhuuu	Sssss	Fffuuu	Shhuuu Shhiii
Tissues	Veins Arteries	Muscles Fascia	Body Hair Skin	Bones Marrow	Tendons Nerves
Senses	Taste	Touch	Smell	Hearing	Sight
Orifices	Tongue	Mouth	Nose	Ears	Eyes
Tastes	Bitter	Sweet Bland	Pungent	Salty	Sour Astringent
Food Examples	Coffee/Tea Asparagus Lettuce Greens	Yams Molasses Oats	Leeks Garlic Cinnamon	Kelp Seaweed Seafood	Lemon Plum Orange Vinegar

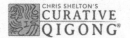

CHAPTER 32

THE FIRE ARCHETYPE

Compass direction: South

Season: Summer

Color: Red

Taste: Bitter

Internal organs: Heart, Small Intestine; Pericardium, Triple Burner

Expressed in: Veins, arteries; tongue

Positive expressions: Joy, clarity, love

Negative emotions: Sadness, confusion, over-excitation, manic behavior

Underlying Principle

The Fire Element is most active in the summer. It represents exuberant activity, warmth, and clarity.

PHYSICAL ATTRIBUTES

Fire people tend to be small in stature with slim hips and shoulders, mobile hands, sparkling eyes, and redness in the throat and neck areas. Lively, cute, and charming, their main goal in life is to play. They love new experiences and excitement, which can predispose them to becoming thrill-seekers.

Fire types bask in the limelight and are generally charismatic, charming, and adept at communication. They are full of ideas but prefer starting to finishing. To a more sedate personality, the Fire person can appear impulsive, changeable, and scattered. The Fire type is normally unconcerned with wealth, yet fond of beauty. They are naturally attuned to rhythm and love to dance to a strong beat. Fire minds can be so active that they never shut down, and this can lead to elaborate and active dreams. A Fire type can illuminate and give comfort in any situation. This archetype tends to walk fast, be very creative, and willingly take on many challenges. They tend to flourish in warmer climates as they dislike wearing much clothing and have a naturally high body temperature.

The Fire Element rules the Heart which, in turn, is considered to rule the expression of all emotions. Even though every organ has its own emotions, the Heart decides whether they will be expressed and to what extent. The Fire Element governs communications of all kinds, especially the use of words spoken verbally or in sign language. Because the Heart controls expression, wrinkles on the face will show how much expression has been demonstrated over time. The ancient Chinese feared Fire because, in excess, it dries up the all-important Yin Essence and wears out the body. However, Fire is also necessary for the enjoyment of life, and containing it too much may be even more harmful. There is a primal human need for expression and enjoyment.

The strength of Fire is shown—and is said to "burn"—in the tips and corners of all the facial features. A pointed chin and sharp tips of the eyebrows, ears, nose, and lips are Fire traits. Fire "burns" particularly in the eyes. The eyes are the facial feature most closely associated with this element. Their brightness and quality reflect the presence of inner spirit, or Shen. The Shen reflects changes in emotion from moment to moment, and how well the nervous system is functioning. From the Shen, you can determine how quick someone's mind is. Babies with bright eyes are recognized as being very intelligent. Because of the complex network of muscles that surround the eyes, they are the most expressive feature on the face and the most easily marked. We learn very early in life how to communicate with our eyes, and they reveal our inner truth.

EMOTIONAL ATTRIBUTES

The two emotions specifically associated with the Heart are joy and sadness. Practitioners of Chinese medicine often speak of "excess joy" being dangerous. I believe this is a mistranslation. What the ancients intended to communicate was that excessive excitement, or mania—not joy—is considered harmful to one's health. Also, somewhat in contradiction to typical interpretations, I consider sadness an emotion of the Heart in addition to the Lungs. Sadness is simply a letdown from the high that Fire lives on. It can be seen as the period between the time when the candle flame blows out and when it is relit. Because the Heart and Lungs are closely connected, sadness can turn into sorrow, a deeper and more long-lasting Lung emotion. Unless resolved, in time, sorrow will turn into grief, the primary emotion of the Lungs.

RECOGNIZING DISHARMONIES IN THE FIRE ELEMENT

Strong Fire

If your score indicates you are primarily a Fire type, look to the Blood, blood vessels, and nervous system for keys to your physical health. A Fire type's most serious health problems are likely to come from inflammation caused by unrestrained Fire and an overactive nervous system; this includes lupus and rheumatoid arthritis. Fire people are also prone to disturbances in speaking and thinking that are caused by the misfiring of the brain and an overactive imagination; these include stuttering, phobias, and mental illnesses. As stated earlier, the Fire Element's primary organ is the Heart, which controls and regulates the expression of all emotions. Suppression of emotions can, therefore, cause problems with the heart, including arrhythmia, tachycardia, and heart disease. When out of balance, Fire types struggle with setting and maintaining boundaries, depleting their energy reserves and leading to exhaustion. With age, Fire people tend to maintain a youthful persona and attempt to continue living an erratic life that ultimately leads to burnout and sadness.

Deficient Fire

Deficiency in an element will also lead to imbalance. People who are deficient in the Fire Element may become prone to heart-related problems, and/or problems within their veins, arteries, or blood.

Achieving Harmony in the Fire Element

To increase the power of the Fire Element in your life, use the color red, angular objects, and anything bright and shiny when decorating your living space. For example, you may want to wear more red clothing and add candles and pictures of fire or buildings with steep roofs (like churches with steeples) to your environment. Pyramid shapes and mountain ranges with steep peaks also support the Fire aspect, as does sleeping with your head in the direction of south.

Conversely, to calm overactive Fire, reduce all of these influences. Also, consider adding calming practices, such as yoga and meditation, to your routine and limiting your social life to allow your internal battery to recharge.

In terms of diet, a Fire person should avoid alcoholic beverages and caffeine, both of which exacerbate the active principle. Adding bitter foods to the diet, particularly those that grow quickly, such as kale, dandelion greens, bitter lettuces (like escarole), and other bitter foods including bitter melon, is very beneficial. This is because the bitter flavor stimulates energy flow in the Heart meridian.

Case History

At a certain point in my life, I knew my Fire Element was deficient in Qi. Several relationships had ended badly. I felt discouraged and frustrated. My Heart center was unwilling to invest in another relationship, yet I craved companionship. To restore my Heart Fire, I changed my living environment and shifted my bed so that, when sleeping, I would be facing south. I bought two red pyramids (a shape that represents Fire) and placed them on the windowsill above the bed. I also added red items to the room's décor, including red candles. The effects were not instant, but within a month or two, I noticed changes. I met more Fire people and felt increasingly optimistic. Ultimately, it was around that time that I met my wife, who is a Fire type.

CHAPTER 33

THE EARTH ARCHETYPE

Compass direction: Central

Season: Late summer/early autumn

Color: Orange, yellow

Taste: Sweet, bland

Internal organs: Spleen, Stomach

Expressed in: Muscles, mouth (lips)

Positive expressions: Serenity, centeredness, peace of mind

Negative emotions: Worry, anxiety

Underlying Principle

The Earth Element is most active in late summer/early autumn. It represents stability, serenity, and warm affection.

PHYSICAL ATTRIBUTES

The major physical signs of Earth are plumpness in the abdominal area, lower cheeks of the face, upper arms, and calves. The Earth archetype may have a darkish complexion, well-developed thighs, and a wide jaw. In particular, Earth types tend to have strong muscles. The Earth person has to watch out for gaining weight, because a large belly and somewhat heavy body type are attributes of Earth.

The facial feature most strongly related to the Earth Element is the mouth, and in particular, the lips. The mouth is the place we take in nourishment, and it is also the most sensual part of the face. The size of the mouth indicates the appetite of a person, not only for food but also for affection, information, things, etc. Therefore, the bigger the mouth, the more a person desires. The mouth is a feature that expresses emotions easily, as in a smile or kiss. It is the second most changeable feature on the face, after the eyes. Most major expressions require movement of the mouth. The mobility of the muscles around the mouth allows people to quickly change its shape in an extraordinary range of movements. For this reason, it reveals much about an individual.

A large mouth demonstrates generosity and the ability to give. Larger mouths belong to people with an abundance of Earth energy. The size of the mouth is measured in relation to the nose. Imagine a triangle starting at the center point in the bridge of the nose and follow the sides of the nose down to the mouth area. The average mouth is the same length as the width at the base of this imaginary triangle. Any mouth that goes beyond this measurement is considered wide. A mouth measuring less than this may be considered small.

To the ancient Chinese, a large mouth was thought to be a fortunate feature. Men with large mouths are supposedly more capable of attracting a good wife. People with large mouths are typically generous and may buy many gifts for those they love, as well as for business associates. They are known to spontaneously give things, even to strangers or new acquaintances. People with average-sized mouths still have generosity but tend to be more particular about to whom and how much they give. Those with small mouths will find it difficult to give unless there is good reason. They are more conditional about giving and may only do so because someone deserves it or they are supposed to; this kind of giving is based more on practicality than the emotion that drives an Earth type.

The size of the lips is also a factor in determining one's type. Fullness of the lips is evaluated based on the fleshiness of the rest of the face. Someone whose face demonstrates Earth qualities, with plump cheeks and a puffy nose will tend to also have bigger lips while those with taut skin and aquiline features will have thinner lips. Exceptions to this are considered "magnified" traits. In general, fuller lips belong to people who are more expressive emotionally. They are considered romantic and sensual as plump lips indicate a desire for pleasure. People with thinner lips are said to be more reserved emotionally, especially if they hold them together in a compressed fashion.

Vertical wrinkles on the philtrum above the upper lip can indicate Earth deficiency, or conditions where a person typically gives more than he/she receives, or has somehow not been nurtured fully throughout their lives. It can also reflect a deficiency in physical nutrition.

EMOTIONAL ATTRIBUTES

Earth people tend to be sedentary; they enjoy sitting. They value comfort, consistency, and pleasure while thoroughly enjoying food and companionship. Earth types are the collectors of the world and love to accumulate both possessions and people. They become very attached to their loved ones and belongings, and are generally considered to be warm and affectionate.

Although not very ambitious, Earth types are known to be calm and centered. Earth represents stability, and the element harmonizes all others. Fairness is a predominant quality of an Earth person. Being highly trustworthy, Earth types make great managers and organizers. At the same time, their focus can be weak, making the handling of multiple tasks quite difficult, often leading to worry. An Earth person is best able to respond to change when it is gradual.

RECOGNIZING DISHARMONIES IN THE EARTH ELEMENT

Strong Earth

When the Earth Element is in excess, there is a strong tendency to overeat and gain weight, often to the point of obesity. Earth people tend to worry and feel excessive sympathy for those they care about, and this can lead them to become overly involved in the lives of others. As Earth types move slowly, they can become "stuck" in their habits, creating cycles and patterns that are hard to shift.

Stagnant Earth

Earth stagnation manifests as a tendency for circulation issues in the lymphatic fluid and blood, when it may pool or coagulate. This causes such problems as varicose veins, blood clots, and hemorrhoids.

Deficient Earth

When the Earth Element is deficient, there will be problems with the stomach and the digestion of food—as well as ideas. Related conditions include anorexia, bulimia, diabetes, and flatulence. Earth deficiency is common when too much nurturing is given to others at the expense of the self. This is thought to be an underlying causative emotional factor in cancer. Movement and change are encouraged for a more balanced Earth Element.

Achieving Harmony in the Earth Element

The colors yellow and orange, as well as earth tones, support the Earth Element. To benefit Earth, hang pictures of flatlands or plains. The Earth Element is represented by architecture that is both flat and square. Having your surroundings made of earth-derived building materials, which include brick, adobe, or even concrete, is positive for supporting Earth.

While Earth types may be attracted to sugars and sweets, they should avoid excessive amounts of simple carbohydrates. Foods that may help uplift fatigue caused by weakness are yams, corn, and certain types of rice. People that need to balance the Earth Element will greatly benefit from Qigong practices that root Qi and those that harmonize the Stomach and Spleen. They will also benefit from hobbies that allow them to regain a sense of being grounded, such as working with clay, gardening, or simply spending time outdoors in nature.

As the sweet flavor is associated with Earth, those deficient in Earth can add more sweet, yellow, or orange foods to their diet and should eat more bland foods, like oatmeal or rice porridge. Conversely, those seeking to harmonize excess Earth should avoid these foods.

CHAPTER 34

THE METAL ARCHETYPE

Compass direction: West

Season: Autumn

Color: White

Taste: Pungent

Internal organs: Lungs, Large Intestine

Expressed in: Body hair, skin

Positive expressions: Courage, righteousness, justice, truth

Negative emotions: Grief, sorrow, sadness, disappointment, shame, and guilt

Underlying Principle

The Metal Element is most active in autumn. It represents the principles of independence, correctness, and sensitivity on all levels.

PHYSICAL ATTRIBUTES

The major physical attributes of Metal include small bones, very fair skin, and aquiline features. While perhaps appearing delicate, Metal types typically have strong bodies with broad, square shoulders. They may walk slowly, pushing their chest out with their shoulders back. In addition to the fine bone structure and a white undertone to the complexion, the facial feature most strongly expressed by the Metal Element is the nose, which will be aquiline or otherwise prominent.

Metal people have very strong immune systems; they can get sick frequently but recover quickly. People who are Metal dominant typically develop skin and respiratory system allergies early in life, including hives, eczema and asthma. Due to their fair skin, Metal types may get sunburned easily and prefer staying indoors. They are more frequently bitten by mosquitoes because of their ability to release a large quantity of carbon dioxide with their out-breath as they detoxify their lungs. Preferring to cocoon in what they consider safe environments with a minimum of dust or clutter, those ruled by the Metal Element display a maximum of beauty and stylish design.

EMOTIONAL ATTRIBUTES

Metal types are typically more mental than physical. They require refinement, cleanliness, tranquility, and space to thrive. Metaphorically, the element encompasses both people who are like raw ore, out of the earth—practical, independent, strong-willed—and people who are like fine, honed steel—elegant, sensitive, and idealistic. Hence, Metal types can love both simplicity and luxury. They are particular, detail-oriented, and perfectionistic. Metal people normally have powerful voices, their lungs being their strongest attribute. They also express their strong voice when aggressively pursuing their goals, displaying their confidence and intuition. The Metal type is as sensitive to dust and clutter as they are to injustice and dishonesty; they demand respect.

In their negative aspect, Metal types are often seen as aloof and distant and, indeed, may isolate themselves, withdrawing from activities and society in general. Yet this can express their need to maintain healthy boundaries, as they are easily overwhelmed. Metal types are prone to health problems involving a violation of their boundaries and/or failure to express their innermost feelings. In Chinese medicine, the emotion of sorrow is typically associated with the Lungs and Metal Element. This can arise from the deepest of sorrows resulting from a separation from those you love, either by death or behavior. The correlations presented here suggest that breathing deeply may be one of the best self-help methods for restoring a balanced view and acceptance of the circumstances causing sorrow.

RECOGNIZING DISHARMONIES IN THE METAL ELEMENT

Strong Metal

When Metal is too strong, a person becomes rigid and inflexible, with emotional as well as physical repercussions; phobias may develop.

Stagnant Metal

Conditions of stagnation include illnesses that occur because of overcrowding and unclean environments, including tuberculosis and leprosy. Excessive accumulation of phlegm that causes chronic coughing and shortness of breath are also associated with Metal stagnation.

Deficient Metal

When people develop allergies later in life, they have usually become Metal deficient. This also applies to those who never had respiratory ailments as children but frequently suffer from them as adults. Other signs of Metal deficiency include the slow healing of skin as well as chronic respiratory and skin conditions, including recurring bronchitis, emphysema, psoriasis and a general weakening of the immune system. A tendency to catch colds or flus easily is also a sign of a weak Metal Element.

Achieving Harmony in the Metal Element

To support the Metal Element, include metal items and furnishings in your life and house. Use the colors white or silver. Decorate your house with arched, curved, or semi-circular furnishings to gather more Metal energy. In architecture, domed metal roofs or primarily metal structures attract Metal energy.

In terms of diet, to increase the Metal Element, include pungent foods that expel pathogens from the body. Examples of these include garlic, ginger, and mint. In addition, all members of the cabbage family, including horseradish, can supply pungent flavor and support the immune system.

CHAPTER 35

THE WATER ARCHETYPE

Compass direction: North

Season: Winter

Color: Black or deep blue

Taste: Salty

Internal organs: Kidneys, Urinary Bladder

Expressed in: Bones, ears, hair, brain, uterus/testicles

Positive expressions: Wisdom, insight

Negative emotions: Fear

Underlying Principle

The Kidneys store your willpower. The Yang aspect of this will is the power to take responsibility for one's life, making decisive efforts and fundamental commitments. The Yin aspect is the recognition that the deepest of forces requires no work. Yin influences the direction in which we move; it can only be seen or noticed when we look back and realize how much we have developed over time. Through the interplay of these two, in the absence of fear, we develop wisdom.

PHYSICAL ATTRIBUTES

The major physical traits of Water are big bones and wide hips. Water people carry weight in their hips and thighs. They often look multiethnic, which gives them an exotic, mysterious, or secretive persona. Water types are prone to shadows around the eyes.

The facial features most strongly related to the Water Element are the ears, forehead, philtrum, chin, and under eye area. The shape, size, and quality of the tissues of the ears are also indicative of the quality and strength of your Qi. A broad, prominent forehead suggests creativity.

EMOTIONAL ATTRIBUTES

Water people are quiet and observant. They are good listeners and give sound advice, because they have innate wisdom. They appear to be easygoing but, when working, are very persistent. Those ruled by Water require a lot of sleep, rest, meditation, or time to just "be." They are strong both physically and emotionally, handling catastrophes and emergencies in a calm manner. Water types need to watch for being too willful or stubborn. Their main health problems come from the frozen state of Water, which encourages the growth of tumors or high blood pressure from a lack of emotional flow.

RECOGNIZING DISHARMONIES IN THE WATER ELEMENT

Strong Water

Strong Water energy usually leads to longevity when life is lived wisely and energy is conserved rather than spent. In western terms, this is often attributed to good genetic stock, which is, indeed, an important factor. Problems arising in the Water Element are typically diagnosed as either stagnant or deficient, but never excess.

Stagnant Water

When Water energy stagnates, it is not accessible or usable. This affects the thinking and is, therefore, implicated in mental illness and depression.

Deficient Water

Deficient Water occurs when the lifestyle is too active and Qi is not replenished. This causes aging and degeneration of the body as well as problems with infertility and impotence. Water deficiency can be seen in the following conditions: loss of bone density, losing teeth, deafness, thinning hair, osteoarthritis, and bladder weakness. Genetic defects are also considered a primary form of Water deficiency.

Achieving Harmony in the Water Element

To enhance the Water Element, use dark blue or black colors and/or round bowl-shaped objects in your décor, as well as fluid shapes and pictures of water—ideally active water, such as waterfalls, rather than placid lakes which can promote stagnation. Also, the addition of a fountain or playing an audio track of flowing water will promote Water energy. In terms of diet, adding dark colored and/or salty foods, such as seaweed, black beans, kidney beans, etc. can be very beneficial as the flavor stimulates flow of energy in the Kidney and Urinary Bladder meridians.

CHAPTER 36

THE WOOD ARCHETYPE

Compass direction: East

Season: Spring

Color: Green

Taste: Sour

Internal organs: Liver, Gallbladder

Expressed in: Tendons, sinews; eyebrows

Positive expressions: Determination, sense of purpose, creativity, kindness

Negative emotions: Anger, frustration, repressed anger, rage

Underlying Principle

The Wood Element is most active in the springtime. It represents growth and awakening. Its nature is expansive, active, and affirmative.

PHYSICAL ATTRIBUTES

The major physical signs of Wood are sinewy tendons and a hard body. Wood people either look like tall trees or short, compact bushes. Their strength is in their ligaments, tendons, and sinews. When irritated, they typically clench their fists. They are likely to have rectangular face shapes and broad shoulders. The facial features most strongly related to the Wood type are the eyebrows and brow bone, which will both be well-defined.

EMOTIONAL ATTRIBUTES

Wood types, like green shoots in springtime, have a strong sense of direction and need to be constantly "doing." They work and play hard. As workers, they can handle tremendous amounts of pressure and strict deadlines. At the same time, like the branches of a tree, Wood types have a tendency to spread themselves too thin in their drive to stay active. Wood people resist aging and fight the weakening of their bodies, trying to maintain their high levels of activity, both physically and emotionally, throughout their lives.

Wood people are very sociable, with good verbal skills and a love of spirited discussion. However, they also tend to have strong tempers and can be quick to take offense or become frustrated, especially when others don't come through with their obligations. They often have difficulty expressing their innermost feelings.

Wood types have very strong livers and enjoy processing toxins, whether emotional, as caused by anger, or chemical, as in drugs and alcohol. However, failure to process these toxins (for example, hanging on to old anger or resentment) can lead to problems, while too much enjoyment can lead a Wood type to addiction.

RECOGNIZING DISHARMONIES IN THE WOOD ELEMENT

Strong Wood

To keep their natural tendencies in positive expression, Wood types need to pay particular attention to their anger and their need to be active. Their rashness can lead to accidents, and they are prone to injuries of overuse, such as strained, pulled, or torn muscles and tendons. According to CCM and Curative Qigong®, severe cases of overuse of the Wood Element can lead to conditions like Parkinson's disease, where movement and coordination is compromised and ultimately impeded. It can also lead to conditions of exhaustion, including chronic fatigue. Addiction is another tendency that Wood types need to be aware of and avoid.

Stagnant Wood

Stagnant Liver Qi and/or Blood are the most prevalent Wood Element imbalances in people living in modern society. This is the underlying physiological condition associated with impatience and frustration, which ultimately lead to such expressions as road rage and aggression. Allowed to develop further, these conditions can implode, leading to depression.

Deficient Wood

Individuals deficient in the Wood Element may be prone to sudden outbursts of anger and problems with the nerves, eyes, and tendons, or they may be prone to depression. Menstrual issues in women may also signal Wood Element deficiency.

Achieving Harmony in the Wood Element

Green, as the color of the Wood Element, can help overcome a deficient Wood state. Things added to your living environment that support the Wood Element include: constructional materials of wood, tall rectangular shapes (such as columns or towers), and living plants. Sleeping with your head in the direction of east will also increase Wood energy.

In terms of diet, the Wood dominant individual should avoid eating foods that are greasy and fried. If prone to anger-related issues, adding sour foods, such as lemons, limes, and vinegar to the diet is beneficial, as the sour flavor stimulates energy flow in the Liver meridian.

Personal Observation

It is the nature of Yang to go to excess. The spring season is at the start of the year, when Yang energy is fresh and just beginning to increase. People of the Wood archetype, as Wood is the element of spring, also tend to go to extremes. Thus, I can often identify a Wood person because they like to have the color green all around them. They will wear green, decorate with green, and even own green cars. This is not always wise if it exacerbates an already excessive situation. However, it is also difficult to tell a Wood person what to do; like those young shoots in springtime, they can be determined and relentless in pursuing their own way.

FIVE ELEMENTS QUESTIONNAIRE

Instructions

Below you will find five sections, entitled "Phases," each with a list of questions. For each question, answer how you are, rather than how you would like to be. If the question sounds a lot like you, choose a +2. If the question sounds somewhat like you, a +1. Select −1 if it does not seem much like you, and a −2 if it is not like you at all. If you don't know or are unsure, use 0.

When you are done, add up the count for each phase and arrange them in order, from highest to lowest. Turn to the answer page in Chapter 37 to learn your predominant (highest score) and weakest (lowest score) element types.

Facial Shape Reference

As you go through the questionnaire for each of the five groups, there will be a question about your facial shape. Use this graphic to decide which facial shape most resembles you:

Face Shapes

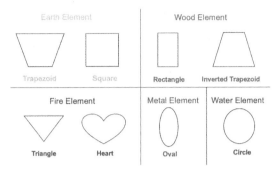

Answer the following questions using this ranking system:

0 for neutral
+1 for somewhat like me
+2 for a lot like me
−1 for not much like me
−2 for not like me at all

Group 1

Do you crave white carbs like pasta and bread? ___
Do you reach for processed sugar when stressed, bored, and/or tired? ___
Is your face predominantly square-shaped? ___
Are your cheeks round and fleshy? ___
Is your jaw strong and angular? ___
Do you have muscular legs and arms? ___
Do you have a potbelly? ___
Do you lose or gain weight easily? ___
Do you often find yourself anxious and worried? ___
Do people ask you to play mediator when there is conflict? ___
Are you known for your good nature, fairness, and generosity? ___
When you're at your best (i.e. well-rested, well-fed, well-meaning), are
    you hopeful for the future? ___
Do people look to you for guidance, advice, and support? ___
Are you recharged by kind, welcoming, and grounded people? ___

Do you love sweets, pastries, and starchy carbohydrates? ____

Do you ruminate and have a tendency to be stubborn? ____

Do you like the colors yellow or orange? ____

Do you become resistant when feeling pressured by others? ____

Can you be stubborn? ____

Do you often eat red meat, bread, potatoes, and pasta? ____

Do you avoid asking for what you want because you don't want to be "difficult" or upset other people? ____

If you disagree with a certain social group or ideology, can you become passive-aggressive or cold? ____

Do you have a low tolerance for rude, self-centered, or ungracious people? ____

When overwhelmed or angry, do you shut down? ____

Are you sometimes accused of giving people the silent treatment? ____

Are you prone to digestive imbalances, like bloating, belching, and flatulence? ____

When under the weather, do you develop sinus issues and become phlegmy? ____

Have you been told you're susceptible to diabetes (e.g., overweight, genetics)? ____

When at a party, do you sometimes feel awkward? ____

Can you be found mixing and mingling with new people? ____

TOTAL: _____

Answer the following questions using this ranking system:

0 for neutral
+1 for somewhat like me
+2 for a lot like me
−1 for not much like me
−2 for not like me at all

Group 2

Do you tend to overeat? ____

When feeling happy or sad, do you crave salty food? ____

Is your face round or oval with full cheeks? ____

Are there sometimes dark circles under your eyes? ____

Are your chin and forehead quite prominent? ____

Do you have "bedroom eyes"? ____

Do you tend to alternate between feeling lonely and feeling loved? ____

Do you sometimes use sex as a way to connect? ____

Are there times when you judge your sex drive as being too strong? ____

Do you sometimes engage in sex because you're feeling lonely or sad? ____

Have you ever used sex as a means of controlling your intimate partner? ____

Do you have a strong sense of discipline and willpower? ____

Do you thrive when setting goals and meeting deadlines? ____

Do you love exceeding your expectations about what you can do, be, and have? ____

When friends want wise, non-judgmental advice, do they come to you? ____

Have you been complimented for your ability to speak hard truths while remaining empathetic and peaceful? ____

Would you describe yourself as vibrant and friendly? ____

Do you easily attract romantic partners and new friends? ____

Do people openly recruit you to be their friend or confidant? ____

Can you hold your temper? ____

Are you impatient with yourself and others? ____

If feeling tired or underappreciated, do you become unfocused, lazy, and/or less ambitious?____

Is your voice especially deep, gravelly, and throaty? ____

Do you love wearing dark clothing (e.g., blue, black)? ____

Have you experienced physical and/or emotional imbalances, such as depression, joint issues, kidney disease, or kidney inflammation (nephritis)? ____

When you're at a party, are you often high, drunk, or overeating? ____

Do you love chatting with vivacious, loud people? ____

At a party, do you have fun but stay alert for potential conflict and drama? ____

If there's drama, do you leave the party immediately? ____

TOTAL: _____

Answer the following questions using this ranking system:

0 for neutral
+1 for somewhat like me
+2 for a lot like me
−1 for not much like me
−2 for not like me at all

Group 3

Do you tend to have a lot of energy followed by burnout and the need to recharge? ____

Do you have either a very low or very high tolerance for spicy foods? ____

Is your face diamond or heart shaped? ____

Do you have sharp angular tips on your eyebrows, eyes, and lips? ____

Is the undertone of your face red? ____

Do you wear your emotions on your sleeve, i.e., people can tell when you're upset? ____

When you walk into a room, do people notice you've arrived? ____

Are you a kinetic, hands-on learner? ____

Are you most confident when communicating with like-minded people? ____

Can you speak in a bold voice and display strong body language? ____

Do you make decisions by listening to your Heart? ____

When nervous about hurting someone's feelings, will you defer to their mood and/or opinions? ____

Do you sometimes tolerate or encourage others' bad behavior? ____

Do you get distracted easily or have a hard time focusing on one thing for a long time? ____

Do people consider you charismatic? ____

Are you fun-loving and a free spirit? ____

Do some people consider you too loud or too bold? ____

Do you trust people easily? ____

Do you consider love more important than riches? ____

Are you a lover of beauty? ____

Do you consider yourself spiritual? ____

Is your tone of voice warm, friendly, and often filled with giggles? ____

Do you love wearing clothing that is red or pink? ____

Do you thrive when feeling loved and cherished by friends and family? ____

Do you tend to have poor boundaries and, as a result, sometimes attract untrustworthy people? ____

Are you prone to giving too much too easily? ____

Could you be more discerning about the people you spend time with (e.g., takers, divas, passive-aggressive types)? ____

Have you experienced physical and/or emotional imbalances, such as mania, depression, exhaustion, arterial problems, or heart issues (e.g., palpitations, high or low blood pressure)? ____

Are you a party person who loves to make people laugh? ____

Do you feel both joy and sorrow more deeply than others? ____

TOTAL: _____

Answer the following questions using this ranking system:

o for neutral
+1 for somewhat like me
+2 for a lot like me
−1 for not much like me
−2 for not like me at all

Group 4

Do you love five-star food and rare delicacies? ____

Are you considered a "foodie" and sometimes a picky eater? ____

Is your face relatively long with a pointed nose? ____

Is your face skinny with prominent bones and delicate features? ____

Do you have thin lips? ____

Is your body long and slender or strong and athletic? ____

Do you walk slowly but with purpose? ____

Have you been accused of having a sharp tongue? ____

When angry or frustrated with others, do you lower your voice? ____

Do you feel sorrowful or sad when alone? ____

Do you use your temper as a shield against feelings of inferiority? ____

Do you consider yourself charming and a natural leader? ____

Do people love being on your "good side" because your temper and/or scorn is notorious? ____

Are you renowned for getting things done? ____

Do you radiate power and status without acting in ways that are loud and proud? ____

Is it rare for you to miss a day of work because of illness? ____

Are you affected by cold and flu season? ____

Is your voice high-pitched? ____

Are you prone to shut down when angry or hurt? ____

Do you sometimes give people the silent treatment? ____

Do you love silk and high-end clothes? ____

Do you like wearing white and gray? ____

Do you dress to impress? ____

Are you susceptible to physical and/or emotional imbalances, such as dry skin (e.g., eczema), lethargy, anemia, low immunity (e.g., seasonal cold and flu), sinus problems and constipation? ____

When you're at a party, are you chatting 1:1 with the smartest person in the room? ____

Do you gravitate toward conversations about the economy, politics, and/or the arts? ____

Do you thrive when you're in a position of high social status? ____

Do people respect your social polish and intellect because you make gatherings more sophisticated and inclusive? ____

Do you enjoy the sound of wind chimes? ____

TOTAL: _____

Answer the following questions using this ranking system:

0 for neutral
+1 for somewhat like me
+2 for a lot like me
−1 for not much like me
−2 for not like me at all

Group 5

Do you like foods that are greasy, fatty, and fried? ____

Do you have a rectangular head and a strong jaw? ____

Do you have a bony forehead and/or protruding brow bone? ____

Do you appear strong and solid irrespective of how tall or short you are? ____

Are you naturally slender? ____

Do you have wide shoulders? ____

Is your back strong and straight? ____

Have you struggled with holding grudges or feelings of anger, rage, and/or depression? _____

Do co-workers consider you a workhorse? ____

Are you able to complete projects quickly and efficiently? ____

Do you feel comfortable when in control and in charge? ____

Do you sometimes attract people who are "followers" and cast themselves as victims? ____

Do problems and obstacles inspire your creativity and resilience? ____

Is creativity one of your strong attributes? ____

Do you enjoy setting goals and completing tasks? ____

Is your tone of voice confident, strong, loud, and clear? ____

Do you often wear clothes that are green? ____

Are you sometimes accused of being a bully? ____

Are you susceptible to physical and/or emotional imbalances, such as migraines, eye problems (e.g., glaucoma, detached retina), menstrual or menopausal issues (e.g., cramping, hot flashes), depression, TMJ, inflammation, and/or body stiffness? ____

Are you prone to digestive imbalances like bloating, belching, and flatulence? ____

When at a party, are you sometimes playing host or hostess even if it's not your party? ____

Do you like working with your hands? ____

Do you fight for the underdog? ____

Are you a thrill seeker? ____

Are you in a leadership position now or do you plan to be soon? ____

Does laziness (both in yourself and in others) irritate you? ____

Is anger your "go-to" emotion? ____

Do you like furniture made of wood? ____

Are you athletic and/or outdoorsy? ____

TOTAL: _____

Putting You and Nature Together: Thriving in a Natural and Elemental Way

Now that you've answered all the questions, compare the tallies for each section. Which set of questions—Group 1, 2, 3, 4, or 5—generated the highest number?

The highest tally is your dominant element, which affects your mind, body, and spirit. The section with the lowest number is your least active element.

It is important to know your primary element typology because a deviation of that type can indicate disease. Likewise, it is also important to be aware of your lowest typology to further help ward off potential diseases.

Knowing and honoring the elements in your nature has the power to supercharge your health and change the trajectory of your life. Congratulations on taking the time to discover the elements of your good nature and your good health!

Results

Group 1: Earth
Group 2: Water
Group 3: Fire
Group 4: Metal
Group 5: Wood

CHAPTER 38

THE EMOTIONAL COMPONENT

You have now seen that Chinese medicine recognizes emotional characteristics as symptoms of energetic imbalances. Disease has physical, mental, and emotional aspects; all are both contributing causes and resulting effects. Interestingly, ancient Chinese texts do not provide techniques for specifically addressing emotional imbalances. This is possibly because, in earlier eras when those texts were written, emotions were not as relatively prominent as they are today. At that time, physical problems were the overriding causes for seeing a doctor. Infectious diseases, accidents, acts of violence, challenges of famine, etc. were the predominant threats to life. Almost no one had a sedentary lifestyle; people had none of the silent stressors that are inescapable aspects of modern life. Instead, most were farmers, spending time alone outdoors and working as their own boss. Life was certainly not perfect, but it was very different.

In today's modern world, as living standards have improved and infectious diseases have come under control, emotions have become much more important in the picture of overall health. Using the correlations inherent in Chinese medicine's descriptions, we now need to consider both physical and mental symptoms in, or contributing to, any condition. For example, you may have high blood pressure or tinnitus; do you also have anxiety, deep-seated sorrow, or perhaps a chronic lack of confidence? To view these as symptoms that you *have*, and not qualities that you *are*, is important for healing. Modern clinical studies have shown that mental and emotional symptoms can not only generate physical symptoms, but also interfere with healing.

Everyone has emotional characteristics, yet none are inherently negative; it is only thinking that makes them so. The natural tendency of the universe is to create harmony. Allowed to flow freely, energy will find a way to express itself in a positive, healthy way. Whatever your elemental archetype or natural inclinations, your traits can be transmuted from ore into gold.

How can you identify emotional imbalances? Generally, you can find them in your actions and reactions to stimuli, situations, and people. They are what make you unhappy, resentful, angry, etc. Any negative thought signals an emotional imbalance; when negative thoughts become a persistent internal voice, they signal a chronic imbalance or, in Chinese medicine terms, a place where your energy is stuck. Such phrases as, "I can't stop thinking about . . . ," "I can't stand . . . ," or "I have never gotten over the loss of . . ." are clues to where your energy is not flowing smoothly. When a healthy person gets the flu, he or she suffers until the immune system takes over and restores harmony. Similarly, when a healthy person experiences an emotional loss or stress, he or she suffers—then recovers. This is the normal process. It's when energy gets stuck that problems arise.

Physical symptoms can also serve as a clue to underlying problems or unresolved emotional issues. It is the typical chicken-egg conundrum; do physical symptoms cause the mental, or vice versa? This cannot be answered. However, the imbalance can be addressed from either side; meaning, in some cases, physical remedies can resolve emotional issues. This is particularly true of Qigong. For example, when you do the Liver Cleansing Exercise, you may suddenly experience a wave of heat leaving the liver area of the body and flowing downward. What was that? You may never know—and it doesn't matter! The body has just healed itself. Be grateful, and move on. Or you may be practicing one of the meditations and suddenly have a new perspective on an old issue, after which it is simply no longer important to you. Case closed.

On the other hand, sometimes physical remedies cannot heal the problem. They may heal it temporarily, but in a day, week, or a month, it comes back, possibly stronger and more intractable than before. Or sometimes a remedy will cure the initial issue, but another pops up, possibly worse than the first. Both of these scenarios suggest the original ailment was not actually cured; the disharmony is still there, perhaps transforming, but not dissolving. In this case, a way of addressing the emotional issue directly is needed.

Modern and ancient techniques offer a number of ways to address, heal, and harmonize emotional energies. These practices are an important complementary support to Qigong in our modern world.

Mindfulness training: This technique has been used for thousands of years to calm the mind. It is derived from the Buddhist practice of Vipassana meditation, popularized by Jon Kabat-Zinn in books and other publications, and taught in many clinics and centers around the world. The idea is that you try to keep your mind-attention on the body. That is all. When your mind strays, you bring it back. The key point, however, is to bring focus back without frustration, discouragement, or any emotional response, whatsoever. You simply resume the practice. During the course of this, all kinds of thoughts may enter your mind; by patiently discarding them, you become able to center the mind in the present moment, rooted in your body.

NLP, or Neuro-Linguistic Programming: I, personally, have used this technique with much success. The thrust of the training is to observe how you are distorting actual reality with your mind—to observe how you create negative, self-destructive attitudes that then generate negative, self-destructive actions. Once aware of these patterns, you can change these attitudes and realize a whole new way of being.

EFT, Emotional Freedom Technique or "Tapping": This is one of the fastest and potentially easiest approaches to resolving emotional issues, requiring no self-discussion or historical analysis. It is based on the use of Chinese medicine's meridians. The procedure is to hold firmly in mind any negative thought or issue that is plaguing you while tapping vigorously 5 or 6 times, sequentially, upon specific points on your head and upper torso. The tapping points are actually acupuncture meridian junctures where emotional energy can get stuck or blocked. Tapping on these points releases the flow of energy. Often what you experience is that a new thought or perspective on your situation spontaneously comes to mind. You then have a choice between the old, painful way of thinking and the new, more balanced, positive way; you will naturally go with the flow into the path of balance, harmony, and joy. The procedure sometimes needs to be repeated, because old habits die hard, but it does usually bring immediate, as well as long-lasting, relief.

Mirror talk: Another very simple technique I have used to address emotional issues and create positive change in my life is to talk to myself in the mirror. This may be uncomfortable, because it's difficult to face yourself; however, with perseverance, the practice can bring unexpected benefits.

In addressing emotional issues, talk to yourself in the mirror with compassion and curiosity. Try to find out what is really going on. What is at the root of the problem? Is it fear? Resentment? Jealousy? Your inner self is doing the best that he/she can; simply try to gain a deeper understanding. It will seem like you become your higher self when talking to your physical self. See what comes up, and allow your higher self to deal with it, keeping in mind your goal of achieving health and harmony.

This technique can also be used to co-create positive attributes with your higher power (whatever you conceive that to be). In co-creating, there are two important principles to keep in mind. First, always talk and think in terms of the positive. For example, if you know you are a controlling person, which is a Liver dysfunction in Chinese medicine, do not say to yourself, "Please help me to not be a controlling person!" Instead say, "I choose to be loving, compassionate, patient, and tolerant" (or whatever the opposite of controlling is for you). In this way, you will affirm and manifest the positive. Second, as you speak to your "self" in the mirror, always use the present tense. Do not say, "I will one day be compassionate" or "I want to be compassionate." Rather, say, "I *am* compassionate!" This is not wishful thinking. In reality, you ARE whatever you want to be. The fact that you can conceive of it means that you have the kernel of that quality already present in yourself; now you want to bring it out and let it flourish.

One of my clients recommends continuing mirror talk until you break into laughter. Laughter is a sure and certain sign of good health. Remember, happiness is your natural state.

Self-Reflection Checklist: In chapter 40, you will find a Self-Reflection Checklist which will further help you address and overcome any negative emotional issues you may have identified to become a more balanced person. It is a grid with a list of statements on the left and checkboxes for each day of the month. Read each statement and give yourself a red mark if you achieved your goal or a black mark if you did not keep an observance. Do this daily or as part of your weekly Renewal of Spirit practices. Using the checklist has two main benefits. First, it should make you more aware of negativity that has slipped into your habitual way of being. It is negativity first in thinking, then in action, which creates disease. Second, it shows you the progress you have made. Acknowledging your progress builds it into your subconscious and promotes further change. At the end of the checklist are blank lines for you to fill in your own statements. You may like to include some physical symptoms, too. It is odd but true that, as people heal, they forget how sick or dis-eased they were in the first place. The Self-Reflection Checklist will provide glowing evidence of your progress.

CHAPTER 39

YIN AND YANG TYPOLOGY QUESTIONNAIRE

Another useful tool (besides the Five Elements questionnaire) is figuring out whether you are a dominant Yin or Yang typology. In chapter 4, I introduced you to Yin and Yang principles. A common misconception is that women are predominantly Yin while men are more Yang. The reason for this misunderstanding is that, traditionally, the feminine is considered Yin and the masculine, Yang. One of the things I love about this philosophy is that nothing is absolute. We can say that nothing is what it appears to be and is, instead, only relative to something else.

One of the diagnostic tools in clinical practice is observing the fingernails. We can tell if someone is more of a Yin or Yang typology by how many of their fingernails have cuticles on them. In-clinic, we call these "moons" because they look like little half-moons! The thumb (generally speaking) will have a moon on the cuticle; showing this will actually tell us the strength of a person's Liver. Therefore, if you have cuticles or moons showing up on two or more fingers of each hand, it indicates you are a Yang type. If there is only the cuticle on the thumb or a tiny moon on both of the index fingers, this generally means you are a Yin type. This chart was given to us at an Infinichi workshop with Dr. Mao Shing Ni at Yo San University in Los Angeles, California. We tested the accuracy of the chart with our Curative

Qigong students in our two-year mastermind program. While learning and applying the section of diagnosis and assessment from palpation, we had our students evaluate each other's fingernails to determine whether or not they were a Yin or Yang type. Then we had them take this questionnaire and cross-reference their fingernail assessment to see if both lined up. I was happy to report that approximately 90 percent of the class's fingernail moons aligned with the questionnaire!

Instructions for Questionnaire

Go through the questionnaire and mark each bullet point you align with. Each is worth one point. This is not a weighted questionnaire. Add up your total scores for the Yin/Venus and Yang/Mars approaches. This will inform you of whether you're a dominant Yin or Yang typology. You can also cross-compare this questionnaire by how many cuticles you see on each of the fingers of both hands. If there are visible cuticles, even if they're small on more than two fingers on each hand, it indicates that you are a Yang type.

Adapted from Infinichi Life Coaching—Dr Mao Shing Ni and Phillip Chrisman

Yin/Venus Approach

- Accepts differences
- Looks at all the various angles of a situation
- Uses creative and diffuse thinking styles
- Finds that logic balances and connects ideas
- Relies on intuition
- Waits for decisions to arise
- Learns through observation and experience
- Values process over product
- Seeks meaning in life
- Values unseen accomplishments, like touching someone's life
- Sees death as part of life
- People-oriented
- Puts others' needs first
- Places relationships before goals
- Believes relationships bring new opportunities

- Experiences love as an energy flow
- Communicates in order to connect
- Connects through sharing thoughts and feelings
- Negotiates to appease others
- Seeks consensus in groups
- Sees power as strength, flexibility, and self-control
- Strives to change oneself
- Finds rank, order, and position unimportant
- Sees responsibility as the ability to respond
- Believes good leaders delegate power and empower others
- Sees healers as those who facilitate the natural healing process
- Believes rules are relative and can be interpreted on a case-by-case basis
- Asserts each person must discover what is right or moral for themselves
- Sees time as organic, adjusting to individual needs and schedules
- Believes natural resources, plants, and animals require attention and protection
- Views science as promoting an understanding of living in harmony with the universe
- Sees maturity as the integration of Yin Yang energies
  Total Yin Score: _____

Yang/Mars Approach

- Judges superior and inferior, right and wrong
- Focuses on relevant data
- Uses direct and logical thinking styles
- Uses reason as a tool to explain and convince
- Relies on the senses to gather information
- Makes decisions quickly and decisively
- Learns through exploration and taking things apart
- Values success and production
- Seeks accomplishments
- Values tangible accomplishments like production and promotions
- Believes accomplishments survive one's death
- Task-oriented

- Puts one's own needs first
- Places goals before relationships
- Believes relationships require sacrifice
- Experiences love as an exchange of gifts
- Communicates in order to exchange ideas
- Connects through sharing activities
- Negotiates to win
- Seeks majority rule
- Sees power as command, control, and influence
- Tries to change others
- Respects rank, order, and position
- Sees responsibility as accountability
- Believes good leaders are a source of strength and authority
- Sees healers as those who identify problems and prescribe remedies
- Believes rules serve the needs of society and should be followed to the letter of the law
- Asserts there are fixed standards of right and wrong toward which everyone should strive
- Sees time as "fixed" and personal schedules should be adjusted for punctuality
- Believes natural resources, plants, and animals exist to serve human needs
- Views science as enabling better control of the universe
- Sees maturity as measured by success, accomplishment, and respect from others

Total Yang Score: _____

CHAPTER 40

SELF-REFLECTION CHECKLIST

Use the Self-Reflection Checklist at the end of the day. Go through each of these observations. If you did well for the day, place a red mark next to the observations, and if you did not meet your goals, use a black mark. You can add other observations at the bottom if your personal goals or challenges are not included here. Do this checklist privately, not around your spouse or significant other. As you fill it out, be kind to yourself and stay open without judgment. The purpose of this checklist is to increase your awareness of your thoughts and actions, which can deviate your Qi and potentially manifest as a disease.

When you do this practice daily, you'll recognize your patterns and gradually be able to change them. If you'd like to print out this checklist, scan the QR code below.

Today I . . .	1	2	3	4	5	6	7	8	9	10	11	12	13	14	15	16	17	18	19	20	21	22	23	24	25	26	27	28	29	30	31
Harmed or threatened to harm someone physically or verbally																															
Lacked trust in/ was suspicious of others																															
Made an unreasonable request/demand																															
Used vulgar language																															
Was critical or judgmental of others																															
Exaggerated, lied, or was otherwise deceitful																															
Broke the trust of another person																															
Disgraced another person																															
Acted vain, conceited, or superior to others																															
Behaved in ways that were overly emotional																															
Let my mood determine my behavior																															

Today I . . .	1	2	3	4	5	6	7	8	9	10	11	12	13	14	15	16	17	18	19	20	21	22	23	24	25	26	27	28	29	30	31
Acted needy or dependent																															
Displayed greedy behavior																															
Resented the success of another																															
Held a grudge																															
Procrastinated																															
Was meddlesome in the affairs of another																															
Was disrespectful of others based on their age																															
Consumed alcohol																															
Engaged in idle talk or gossip																															
Expressed anger in word or deed																															
Behaved out of jealousy																															
Engaged in argumentative behavior																															
Complained about my life, the weather, etc.																															
Sought revenge																															

Today I . . .	1	2	3	4	5	6	7	8	9	10	11	12	13	14	15	16	17	18	19	20	21	22	23	24	25	26	27	28	29	30	31
Blamed others for my own irresponsibility																															
Engaged in bias/ prejudice																															
Ignored an important principle and instead focused something of minor importance to soothe my ego																															
Arrived late to my destination																															
Kept a dirty, cluttered environment																															
Behaved in reckless or irresponsible ways																															
Overindulged (in anything)																															
Felt lazy and did not put in much effort																															
Was wasteful of time, money, or energy																															
Did not follow a proper diet																															
Was unmotivated in my spiritual cultivation																															

Today I . . .	1	2	3	4	5	6	7	8	9	10	11	12	13	14	15	16	17	18	19	20	21	22	23	24	25	26	27	28	29	30	31
Displayed a lack of organization																															
Behaved in ways that are unreasonable or stubborn																															
Engaged in staring at or watching other people																															
Became discouraged when I failed to do what I know is right																															
Felt depressed when deservedly disgraced																															
Praised another person																															
Outwardly expressed my values																															
Forgave someone for their wrongdoing																															
Showed patience																															
Did my best																															
Became discouraged after failing to keep one of these observances																															

⬚ **CHAPTER 41** ⬚

CONCLUSION

You have now finished the course. You have learned four general meditations for keeping your body in balance: The White Pearl, Center and Balance, and Microcosmic/Macrocosmic Orbit Meditations. In addition, you have learned a physical exercise and sound to harmonize the functions of the Yin organ associated with each of the Five Elements, namely, the Heart, Spleen, Lung, Kidneys, and Liver. You are now familiar with Five Elements Principles and the associations with all phenomena in the cosmos, from seasons and compass directions to colors and shapes. You also have tools to work with the emotional components of your health. In other words, you have a firm foundation in understanding how you and other human beings work on an energetic level, and how health is a dynamic balance, affected by emotions, food, and our environment. You can now experience how the human body is a part of the universe. Qi is expressed in everything and nothing (no-thing). Your task now is to apply what you have learned and to continue refining your own true nature.

■ ■ ■

RECOMMENDED READING
AND REFERENCES

I Ching: The Book of Changes and the Unchanging Truth, by Hua-Ching Ni, Seven Star Communications.

Live Your Ultimate Life, Ancient Wisdom to Harness Success, Health and Happiness, by Dr. Mao Shing Ni, Tao of Wellness Press.

The Web That Has No Weaver, Understanding Chinese Medicine, by Ted J. Kaptchuk, O.M.D., Contemporary Publishing Group, Inc.

The Foundations of Chinese Medicine, A Comprehensive Text for Acupuncturists and Herbalists, by Giovanni Maciocia, Churchill Livingstone.

Workbook for Spiritual Development, by Hua Ching Ni, Tao of Wellness Press.

Chinese Medical Qigong Therapy: A Comprehensive Clinical Text, by Jerry Alan Johnson, The International Institute of Medical Qigong.

The Essence of Internal Martial Arts Volumes 1 and 2, Esoteric Fighting Techniques and Healing Methods, by Jerry Alan Johnson, Ching Lien Healing Arts Center.

Tao, The Subtle Universal Law & The Integral Way of Life, by Hua Ching Ni, Tao of Wellness Press.

Face Reading in Chinese Medicine, by Lillian Bridges, Churchill Livingstone.